Martial Arts Injuries

PREVENTION AND MANAGEMENT

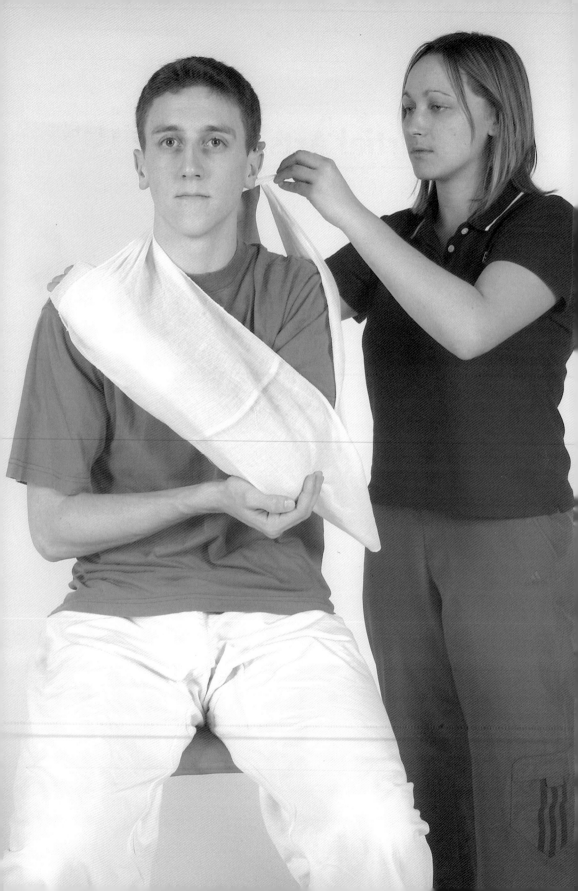

Martial Arts Injuries

PREVENTION AND MANAGEMENT

Neil Barua and Andy Roosen

THE CROWOOD PRESS

First published in 2005 by
The Crowood Press Ltd
Ramsbury, Marlborough
Wiltshire SN8 2HR

www.crowood.com

British Library Cataloguing-in-Publication Data
A catalogue record for this book is available from the British Library.

ISBN 1 86126 732 0

Disclaimer
Please note that the authors and the publisher of this book do not accept any
responsibility whatsoever for any error or omission, nor any loss, injury,
damage, adverse outcome or liability suffered as a result of the information
contained in this book, or reliance upon it. Since martial arts can be dangerous
and could involve physical activities that are too strenuous for some individuals
to engage in safely, it is essential that a doctor be consulted before undertaking
martial arts training.

Throughout this book 'he' 'him', 'his', etc., are used as neutral pronouns and as
such refer to both males and females.

Illustration credits
Line drawings by Keith Field

Typeset by Focus Publishing, 11a St Botolph's Road, Sevenoaks, Kent
TN13 3AJ

Printed and bound in Great Britain by Biddles Ltd, King's Lynn

Contents

Dedication

Neil: For my Mum and Dad – thanks for your guidance and encouragement.

Andy: I would like to dedicate this book to my late mother, Anne Roosen-Verheye, and to my father Mathieu Roosen – thank you always.

Acknowledgements

The authors would like to thank all the people who played a part in the creation of this book, particularly Angela Dobson-Riley, who took all the photographs, and Louise Holden, Abigail Gibson, David Goodacre and Kristian Spoerer, who appeared in the photographs and gave helpful photographic advice. Thank you, also, to Dr Robert Neville for all his editorial comments.

A special thank you goes to Professor Stephen Chan for providing the Foreword, as well as kind advice throughout the project. The authors would also like to thank the martial artists who provided them with the necessary insight into, and feedback on, their training, competition and injuries.

Neil would especially like to thank his Mum, Dad and Amanda for their help and support. Andy would especially like to thank his wife Manu for all her love and support.

Foreword

It is my very great pleasure to write a foreword to this book. I have known and trained with both the authors over a number of years. I cannot think of any others more qualified to write about martial arts injuries than these two fine karate exponents, who also hold academic credentials of a high order directly related to the topic of this book.

The martial arts are frequently misunderstood. Although they are imbued with oriental philosophies, they are not mystical and magical creations. They do not give the superhuman abilities depicted in the films. Instead, they depend on the body being able to move according to physiological principles that are common to all people – oriental, black or white – and they do not prevent injuries. As in any contact sport, injuries are unavoidable, even if their occurence can be minimized by careful and scientific training. Just as it is now possible to plan training regimes that are safer than those of antiquity, so it is also possible and desirable to be able scientifically to treat those injuries that do occur.

The great value of this book is that it covers, comprehensively, not only the treatment of injuries but their prevention. The response to injury is not something mechanical. It relies upon an understanding of how the body works. This book introduces the workings of the body, both its parts and how the parts move in a system. Understanding the system helps the planning of good and safe training that reduces the chance of injury, and leads to proper response when injury does occur.

The book begins with a brief history of the oriental martial arts, and moves to the modern class format in which most students learn these arts. It is a far remove from the legends of the old Shaolin temples but, even there, the monks were required to learn as much about healing as they knew about fighting. The balanced person, in Chinese, Japanese and Korean philosophies, knows how to heal as well as to fight, and knows how to write as well as to struggle in an arena. The authors, in writing this book so well, have tried to live up to an ideal and have tried to help us by way of both instruction and example.

Stephen Chan
8 dan Hanshi in Shorin ryu karate
Professor in the University of London
Dean in the School of Oriental and African Studies

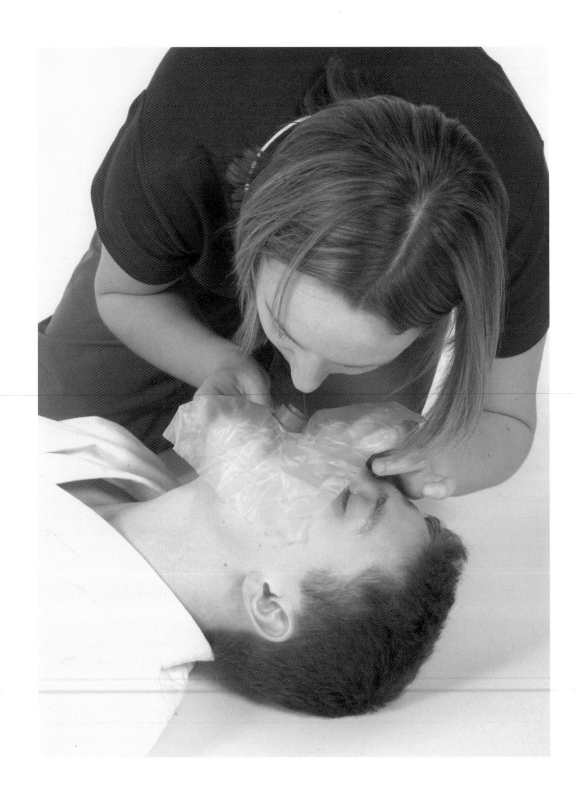

1 Introduction

About This Book

This work is intended to provide the martial arts instructor and practitioner with a tool with which to analyse and reduce the medical risks involved in martial arts training. It presents information to enable the instructor to refine his approach to organizing the structure of sessions. Suggestions on how to prevent injuries are given, common causes of injuries are categorized and outlined, and guidelines on how to treat the most common injuries in martial arts are provided. The selection of the injuries to be discussed has been based partly on our own personal experiences, where we have found them to be the most common, and partly on a survey completed by a number of practitioners across various martial arts.

The first part of the text (Chapters 1, 2 and 3) concentrates on providing a theoretical background to the prevention of injuries in martial arts. The second part (Chapters 4 to 10) is intended to act as a quick reference guide, with each chapter focusing on different types of injuries on various locations on the body. A martial arts instructor or practitioner can quickly find his way to a particular theme or injury and read about how to deal with a casualty.

A Brief History of Modern Martial Arts

As the martial arts continue to become more and more popular, the variety of the activities involved is developing rapidly, and participation in those activities is increasing. But how did the martial arts – in the most literal sense of the term, 'war arts' or 'combat arts' – develop into the modern formats of martial arts today?

Early 'intelligent' man was a hunter and gatherer, living in small social groups. His lifestyle was nomadic, following prey to feed the group, and it was only a matter of time before one group would encounter a rival group. Competing over the same resource, men would have been forced to use their hunting and killing skills to defeat their rivals. Later, as the main means of food provision changed from hunting and gathering to farming, control over areas of land became more important. Groups would venture to steal land from other groups and man would seek to defend his land from his rivals. Presumably, in order to do this effectively, the members of the group would have been taught and trained to fight together, and this is probably the first manifestation of

---

Martial Arts Today

Martial arts have evolved through the ages from a method of combat instruction to an excellent form of physical activity, recreation and sport. It is this development to a modern class system that necessitates a closer look at the methodology of instruction and training, so that injuries can be prevented and treated.

the teaching of a structured way of combat. It is reasonable to assume that any fighting and defence systems developed subsequently had their roots here.

The origin of what are today called martial arts must lie with trained professional warriors, competent in combat systems. Changes in society led to a metamorphosis in the martial arts, from a combat system to a sport-orientated system. The reason for this is simple. In the days before modern weaponry and the definition and enforcement of laws and regulations, the close-range combat arts had more weight for warfare and self-defence than they have today. In order for the martial arts to survive the changes in society, their emphasis also had to change.

Partly due to historic and nationalistic tendencies that arose in the late nineteenth and early twentieth centuries, many of the arts were formalized. A ranking system was incorporated and this brought with it a competitive aspect. Skill was measured against pre-set requirements and sparring and partner drills were inherently present. As this evolution continued, many different rule systems were created for formalized competitions relating to various aspects of a particular art and/or discipline. Many of the arts were introduced to the world due to the two world wars and subsequent wars on the Asian continent, and their rules and ranking systems were spread worldwide, leading to the modern martial arts class set-up.

As there are changes in the societies practising these arts, so the martial arts themselves undergo change. Like an evolving living organism, they lose aspects which are no longer needed, and acquire new features which are necessary to their survival.

With the modern set-up of classes and the popularity of competition, there comes an inherent risk of injuries. The aim of this work is not only to illustrate what those risks are and how they come about, but also to help avoid and reduce injuries and provide methods of treating them.

Types of Training in Modern Martial Arts

When examining how injuries occur in modern training, it is generally reasonable to say that they are due to a force being applied to a part of the body that cannot withstand or handle the magnitude of that force. Different kinds of forces can be encountered in different ways in the course of a typical martial arts class.

Instruction in the martial arts consists of a spectrum of types of training with varying emphasis. This spectrum includes training forms, or patterns and sets, as well as partner exercises and sparring, or fighting. In terms of injuries and injury risk, it is possible to differentiate between the following two types of training within a class format: individual practice which does not require a partner, and practice with a partner. Certain types of injury will be more common to individual training and others will be more common to partner-assisted training. The most obvious difference is that, in partner-assisted training, an individual needs to cope with forces and powers generated outside of his own body.

Injuries that occur in individual practice can also occur when doing partner practice. The opposite, however, is much less likely. For example, a person can pull or strain a muscle doing a set of moves on his own into the empty air, but can also suffer that same injury when trying to do the moves on a partner. However, any impact injuries caused by moves applied by a partner or on to a partner cannot occur when practising alone. A possible exception to impact injuries occurring in individual training is when training with weapons or with other accessories such as bags, a makiwara, or a wooden dummy. Additionally, individual break-fall practice could lead to impact injuries.

Forces At Work

Basic Understanding of Forces

During training in martial arts, it is useful to have a basic understanding of forces and how they can work on a body, and how they can therefore cause injury during practice. Fundamental physical laws will apply here.

Newton's First Law of Motion, or the Law of Inertia, describes how objects are reluctant to move, or change their speed, if they are moving. If they are at rest, they will remain at rest or, if they are in motion, they will continue to move at their current speed. The only way to change this is to apply a force to the object. The heavier an object is, the higher its inertia. In the context of martial arts, this means that the heavier a person (or object) is, the more difficult it is to move him (or it), and the greater the force required to do it.

Newton's Second Law of Motion, or the Law of Acceleration, describes how the momentum of an object can be changed. The more weight or speed a body possesses, the higher its momentum is. A lighter body can, however, still have the same momentum as a heavier one. If one person weighs half as much as somebody else, but moves twice as fast, then both have the same momentum. If the speed of the lighter person is even higher, he will have more momentum than the heavier person. Therefore, momentum is a measure of the amount of motion a body possesses. In simple terms, it defines how fast a body of a certain weight is moving.

In martial arts, as in most dynamics for sports, the weight of an object or person stays the same. Any changes in momentum are therefore due to changes in velocity. So, in this framework, momentum is defined by how fast a body (or body part) of a certain weight is moving. In order to change the velocity of a body, a force needs to be applied to it over a certain time period. How much a body's velocity and momentum are changed depends on the size of the force applied to it. If you want to speed the body up, you need to push it along more; if you want to slow it down, you need to hold it back. The harder you try to push it along, the quicker the velocity and momentum will increase. The more you hold it back, the quicker the velocity and momentum will reduce. The change in velocity is called acceleration if the body's speed is increased, or deceleration if the body's speed is decreased.

For example, if the arm is held in a guard position, it is reluctant to move on its own. A force needs to be applied to it so it will execute a punch. The necessary muscles contract so that the hand is accelerated towards the target and its momentum increases. In order to slow the punch down so it comes to a stop, different muscles apply another force. The hand decelerates and its momentum is reduced.

Newton's Third Law of Motion or the Law of Reaction states that to every action there is an equal but opposite reaction. Applying a force to an object will result in a force of the same magnitude being applied in the opposite direction.

The above three laws are applicable to linear movement, or movement in a straight line. There is another type of movement that needs to be considered, namely rotation, or movement in a circular fashion. The concepts of linear and circular movement, however, are the same. This means that Newton's Laws can be translated for circular motion as well, but a number of new terms need to be introduced. Just as an object can

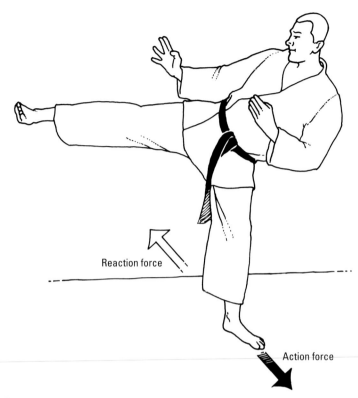

Reaction force

Action force

The nature of reaction force.

possess momentum if it moves in a linear way, or straight, it can possess 'angular momentum' when it moves in a circular way. (The term angular momentum simply relates to a circular motion rather than a linear motion.) Just as a force causes the linear motion of an object – in other words, movement in a straight line – angular force, or 'torque', causes rotational motion of an object (in other words, movement in a circle).

Newton's First Angular Law, or the Conservation of Angular Momentum, states that an object shall remain still or continue to rotate at the same speed, unless an external torque is applied to it. A body's reluctance to changing its rotational motion is called the Moment of Inertia.

Newton's Second Angular Law defines angular force, or torque. It states that the degree to which the angular momentum of an object changes depends on the size of the torque causing the change.

Newton's Third Angular Law is analogous to his third Law of Motion and states that for every action torque there is an equal but opposite reaction torque.

How Do Forces Cause Injury?
Having established that typical martial arts training is conducted either individually or with a partner, it is possible to draw the basic conclusion that, in movement or main-taining posture, forces and torques are at work. These forces and torques work on our own body, on a partner's body, or on other objects. They are generated either by us or by our training partner.

Basically, there are three categories of causes of injury:

Category 1: Injury caused by (a summation of) forces and/or torques generated by the individual in or on his own body.

Category 2: Injury caused by (a summation of) forces and/or torques generated by the individual on another person's body (or object). This implies that the reaction forces and/or torques are causing the injury.

Category 3: Injury caused by (a summation of) forces and/or torques generated by another person on the individual's body.

The forces or torques that come into play may be a summation of forces and/or torques. For example, a Category 3 injury may occur when one individual is applying force to the other, trying to counter the force already being applied; this is typical in wrestling when resisting an attempt to lock a joint. The torque resulting from the force trying to apply the lock (F_A) may be slightly greater than the torque resulting from the force resisting the lock (F_R). Therefore, the resulting torque (T_{Tot}), which is the summation of T_R and T_A, bearing in mind their different direction, as per Category 3, could cause injury. Similar examples can be found for summation forces for Category 1 and 2 causes.

Category 1 and 2 injuries are caused *actively* – forces generated by the individual himself, whether working internally or externally, cause the injury. It is the action of the individual that is directly responsible for the resulting force(s) that cause(s) injury. Category 3 injuries are caused *passively* – an external force applied on the individual causes the injury. The action of another party, such as a training partner or opponent, is responsible for creating the force(s) that result(s) in injury.

Based on the three categories of causes, it is possible to distinguish two major types of injury: *overload* and *over-use*.

The first type of injury is due to an overload of energy and injuries classified within this acute type are either *extrinsic* or *intrinsic*. In an extrinsic injury the force causing the injury originates from outside the individual's body. In the case of an intrinsic injury the force causing the injury originates from inside the individual's body.

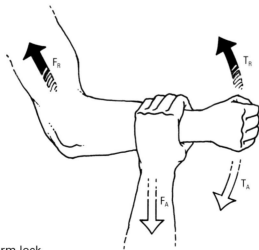

Forces at work in an arm lock.

13

Extrinsic overload injuries occur directly. An excessive force is applied from outside the individual's body and the injury occurs acutely. Category 3 injuries are typically extrinsic injuries.

Intrinsic overload injuries also occur directly, but the damaging force is applied from inside the body. The action of the individual causes the injury. Category 1 injuries are typically intrinsic injuries.

Category 2 involves a force generated from an intrinsic location meeting a reaction force on impact. Although the reaction force could be considered to be extrinsic, it would not exist without the intrinsic action force, and Category 2 injuries are therefore considered to be intrinsic.

(The definition used here for extrinsic and intrinsic applies to overload injuries only. The classification 'extrinsic' or 'intrinsic' is related to the location on the body where the force that causes the injury originates. We do not adopt the definition used by some that an extrinsic cause of injury is synonymous with what is defined here as an overload injury. In this case, there is no reference to the location of the originating force. This alternative definition also says that an intrinsic cause is synonymous with what has been referred to here as an over-use injury.)

The second type of injury is caused by over-use. Occurring indirectly, over-use injuries are of a chronic nature and happen over a period of time as a small force is applied again and again on the same site.

They can be due to bad execution of technique, inflammation or deterioration of tissue due to stress, and/or over-use, and typically involve tendon damage. Certain injuries classed as Category 1 or Category 3 can be over-use injuries.

Examples of Various Types of Injury

One injury belonging to Category 1 would be a strained hamstring resulting from the execution of a kick. This is an acute, intrinsic overload injury. Another example of a Category 1 injury could be an inflamed knee joint caused by incorrect technique in particular movements; this can occur when moving in front stances, or when pivoting on the standing leg to do round-house kicking. This would be a chronic over-use injury.

Impact injuries are typical examples belonging to Category 2. The wrist may be strained and give way under the pressure when an object or an opponent is punched. When kicking, bruising may develop on the instep of the foot after impacting the target. These are acute, intrinsic overload injuries.

An example of a Category 3 injury could be a broken rib after being hit by an opponent, or a strained neck after being held in a headlock. These are acute, extrinsic overload injuries. If a joint becomes inflamed following the repeated application of certain locks to it by a training partner (for example, a wrist lock), a chronic over-use injury may develop.

2 Principles of Injury Prevention I – Preparing to Train

In general, the risk of injury can be reduced by the following measures:

- avoiding training errors;
- eliminating unsafe practice;
- adequate physical conditioning;
- correct alignment of the body.

Physical Conditioning

Physical conditioning is important in order to keep the body in a state which enables it to do the amount of exercise that is demanded of it. It is important to be able to distinguish between the different purposes of types of exercises. One purpose of exercise is to maintain the body's current condition. The second purpose is to enhance the body's condition and prepare it for more difficult exercises; these more demanding exercises can only be done after certain strengthening.

Ensuring that the body is in a condition in which it can perform the required workload will reduce the risk of injury. A martial arts instructor therefore needs to be able to analyse the current fitness level – strength, aerobic capacity and flexibility – of an individual and establish how to improve it for the tasks at hand. To this end, it may be useful to design specific classes in which only conditioning exercises are done. For example, if three martial arts sessions are taught in a week, one of them should be a conditioning class. The exercises undertaken in these classes vary from general conditioning exercises to conditioning exercises that are specific to martial arts. This approach can be more effective than trying to include the conditioning work that is required to maintain the body in classes that should focus on technical training. Separating the themes of the classes can be best for improving the students' fitness as well as their technical skill, as they are able to focus on each aspect separately.

If this approach is not feasible, and both aspects need to be covered in one session, technique training should always be done before conditioning. The conditioning work will tire the students too much if it is done before technique training, and they are likely to perform poorly when being taught technique.

The martial arts training schedule that is devised by the instructor should be progressive, and in order to achieve this it is helpful to have an understanding of the concept of 'physical work capacity' and of how the body develops power.

Physical Work Capacity

'Physical work capacity' (PWC) or physical fitness has two major contributory factors:

genetic endowment (which is outside the control of the individual) and acquired function or training effect. The second factor is within the control of the individual as it is affected by the type of training that is done; it relates to matters such as strength, speed and flexibility, and the results include power and technique.

PWC can be divided into two major aspects: the work performed and the power generated. Both of these aspects are dependent on the individual's aerobic and anaerobic capacity. The aerobic capacity means the amount of energy that can be generated by burning energy-storing molecules using oxygen. Consequently, anaerobic capacity means the amount of energy that can be generated by burning energy-storing molecules without using oxygen. Anaerobic metabolism is a fast self-limiting process. The anaerobic capacity of any individual is therefore very restricted.

It is important to know that PWC is dominated by the aerobic component, and that the fuel and oxygen availability is therefore crucial. An explanation of how both methods of metabolism operate will illustrate the theory.

Adenosine triphosphate (ATP) is a chemical that holds energy. Muscles can release this energy and use it to perform mechanical work. ATP is stored in very limited quantities in muscles. It can also be generated by breaking down other chemicals. In the very short term creatine phosphate (CP), which is also stored in the muscles, is broken down to supply more ATP. The energy supplied using this method is only sufficient for three to five seconds of maximal work. When this initial store of energy runs out, the muscle cell will start breaking down muscle glycogen (chains of sugar molecules stored in muscle tissue) to generate more ATP and, therefore, more energy to perform work. This process happens without using oxygen

(anaerobically) and will produce lactic acid in the muscle. This method of supplying the muscle with energy enables the martial artist to work at a high rate for a short period. It will fuel maximal work lasting two to three minutes.

In the long term, energy will be produced by metabolizing a range of fuels using oxygen. This is called aerobic metabolism. Oxygen breathed in from the air is transported in the red blood cells. Upon reaching the exercising muscle cell, the red blood cells release the oxygen and take the carbon dioxide produced, which is transported back to the lungs and is exhaled. The primary sources of fuel include muscle glycogen, blood glucose (sugar molecules in the bloodstream), plasma free fatty acids (fat molecules in the blood stream) and intramuscular fat (fat stores between muscles). All these molecules are broken down using oxygen within the muscle cell. This way, no lactic acid is produced. The process is slower and it may take up to two to three minutes to get going and supply the energy needed by a muscle cell. Aerobic metabolism is the primary source of energy for maximal work lasting more than two to three minutes and for all types of sub-maximal work.

The aerobic metabolism of one glucose molecule produces nineteen times as much energy as the anaerobic metabolism of the same molecule. The metabolism of fatty acids, which can only occur aerobically, yields even more energy, depending on the length and structure of the chain of the fatty acid.

The point at which an individual switches from aerobic metabolism into anaerobic metabolism is called the 'anaerobic threshold'. Once over this threshold, lactic acid will be produced as part of the metabolism, which will cause the blood and muscle tissue to become more acidic. This in turn causes muscle contraction and fuel metabolism to reduce and eventually cease, until the correct acidity for their optimum functioning has been restored.

If an individual reaches his anaerobic threshold at quite low levels of exercise and is not allowed to recover, fatigue will set in and injuries can occur. Targeted training will allow individuals to move their anaerobic threshold to a higher level.

Proper conditioning for a martial art will consist of a combination of strength, aerobic, flexibility and power training (*see* below), along with co-ordination training specific to the art. In martial arts classes, the aerobic capacity will play a big part, due to the duration of classes. However, anaerobic metabolism becomes very important in explosive power techniques and also in competition bouts, as sudden energy bursts are required and these are powered anaerobically. The importance of anaerobic fitness in a particular martial art will be determined by factors such as the competition rules and the timeframe of a match or round. The competition training undertaken should reflect these factors.

A martial arts instructor must allow the students to build up their aerobic capacity and not simply keep training within the anaerobic range. If an individual can achieve a particular workload aerobically rather than anaerobically, he will be able to continue more efficiently. Due to the nature of martial arts, it is important also to train within the anaerobic range, as this is an inherent part of the martial arts training routine and matching. It will allow the individual to improve mechanisms to cope with the build-up of lactic acid and optimize ways of removing lactic acid from muscle. During hard anaerobic bouts of training, there must be room for easy loads in between, in order to allow the body to remove accumulated lactic acid. In this way, training can continue without fatigue setting in.

Developing Power

Power is determined by the factors of strength, speed and flexibility, which all go hand in hand with technique. Manuals other than this one will give more detail on how to get stronger, faster and fitter, but some of the theory is relevant here, as it relates to the understanding of injury prevention. If the exercised muscles are in adequate condition, the chances of injuring them are reduced. In addition, since martial arts training involves impact (punches, kicks, throws), the presence of some muscle tissue helps in absorbing the blow, so that the underlying tissues are not damaged. Training and conditioning in martial arts must meet certain requirements in order to be effective. Specific training is advantageous and can affect muscle development in certain ways.

It is important to realize that the response to training is specific – in simple terms, you get good at what you practise. Training regimes that are designed to strengthen muscles for a certain purpose should relate not only to the exercising muscle, but also to the movement pattern for which they are intended. The type of adaptation that occurs in the body as a result of training is specific to the type of training undertaken. It is therefore important for a martial arts instructor to analyse the techniques that are required, and to design and recommend exercises that will enhance, strengthen and, to a certain extent, mimic those techniques. Some of these exercises can be included in the conditioning classes.

The last point to make about muscle strengthening – indeed, any training – is that it is reversible. If the muscles are not maintained properly and progressively, the effects of training will undo themselves. If the activity is restarted after a long break, at the same level at which it was abandoned, this could lead to injury. Furthermore, once a long-term training regime is stopped, the maximal oxygen uptake will drop immediately due to a decrease in stroke volume (amount of blood moved by the heart per heartbeat), and, in the long term, due to a reduction in oxygen uptake from the blood. This will affect the anaerobic threshold as less oxygen is available to be burned. A reduction in training, however, has minimal effect on the maximal oxygen uptake as long as the intensity of training is maintained at a high level.

In relation to this last point, it is worthwhile noting that, as the body adapts to any new workload, performance is likely to drop until coping mechanisms are in place. This means that, when the intensity of the sessions is increased, the students will display a drop in performance until they have established a way of handling the new workload. During this period, extra care must be taken to avoid injury.

Muscle Contractions

Muscles can contract in several ways. The *isotonic contraction* involves the muscle developing tension to overcome a resistance in order to move a body part. Typically, this happens in lifting activities. In martial arts activities, this could be involved in a shoulder or hip throw or a sweep.

In an *isometric contraction*, the muscle contracts without changing its length. This happens when trying to move or lift an immovable object, or when trying to resist being moved. One example in martial arts is during wrestling or grappling. Both opponents are trying to move (a body part

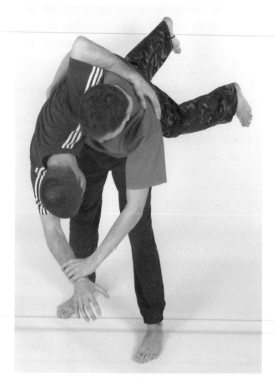

Isotonic contractions in a hip throw.

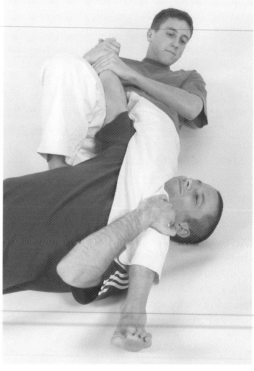

Isometric contractions in wrestling.

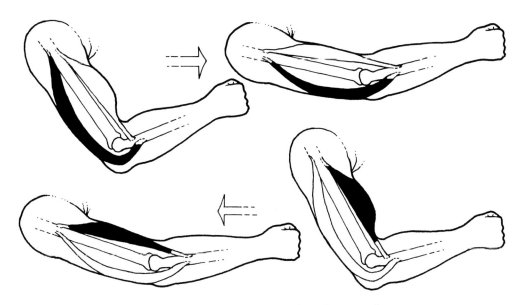

Concentric (in black) and eccentric (in white) contractions in a punch.

of) each other but the resistance cannot be overcome. This is also called a *static contraction*. The risk of injury is quite high in this type of contraction. For example, an individual resists the attempt of an opponent putting on a lock and tries to bend the arm. The opponent, however, is steadily winning the battle of strength and is slowly straightening the arm. If not properly conditioned, the muscle fibres of the resisting muscles can be damaged quite easily.

Concentric and *eccentric* contractions are each other's opposites. The concentric contraction brings the two ends of a muscle closer together and shortens the muscle, whereas an eccentric contraction moves them further apart in a controlled manner, lengthening the muscle. Eccentric contraction is associated with a muscle resisting a movement and slowing it down. However, it is important to point out that muscles always work in pairs. The muscle working with the movement is the *agonist*, and contracts concentrically to move the joint in the desired way. A concentric contraction is required for joint movement to be rapid, and for it to be in the opposite direction of another force. The muscle stopping this action is the *antagonist*, which will contract eccentrically to limit the movement. An eccentric contraction controls the speed of movement caused by another force.

If the antagonist is not strong enough to balance the action of the agonist, acute or chronic injuries can occur.

A movement analysis of a simple punch will illustrate the changing roles of the muscles involved. On punching the hand out, the triceps muscles will be the agonists. They will contract concentrically as the triceps shorten, moving the upper and lower arm apart around the elbow joint. The biceps muscles are the antagonists. They are resisting the upper and lower arm moving away from each other by contracting eccentrically, and lengthening. On retraction of the fist, both muscle groups change roles. This time the biceps muscles are the agonists, which, as they contract concentrically, dominate the movement, while the

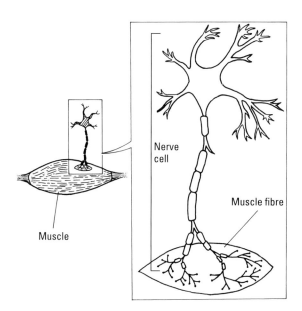

A motor unit.

eccentric contraction of the triceps muscles resists the movement.

It is important to note, however, that, since the martial artist is trying to punch and kick as quickly as possible in most cases, the eccentric contraction is far less than the concentric contraction. Only moves done by tensing the muscles during movement will significantly work the eccentric side. (Many martial arts teach forms that are executed slowly and under tension. These work the concentric as well as the eccentric contractions of the muscles.)

The last type of contraction is *isokinetic*. This is a contraction at constant speed through the whole range of motion. Generally, this can be done only when using purpose-designed equipment, which automatically varies the resistance.

Muscles are made up of motor units, consisting of a nerve cell or neurone and the muscle fibre it controls. As a muscle contracts, it recruits motor units. The strength of a contraction depends on the amount of motor units that have been 'switched on'. Each individual motor unit is subject to an 'all or nothing' response; They are either working or they are not.

The speed of a muscular contraction is determined by the ratio of types of muscle fibres within the muscle. There are three major types:

Type 1: the slow-twitch muscle fibre contracts and relaxes slowly but is resistant to fatigue and well suited for endurance activities.

Type 2a: the fast-twitch muscle fibre that uses oxygen to burn sugars in order to produce the energy needed has less endurance than the Type 1 fibre, but more than the Type 2b fibre (*see* below). Both Type 2s are twice as fast as Type 1 fibre in their contraction.

Type 2b: the fast-twitch muscle fibre that does not use use oxygen to burn sugar and has, therefore, the least endurance due to lactic acid production. However, it does produce the most force.

An individual is unable voluntarily to influence the pattern of fibre recruitment, which occurs in the following sequence: 1, 2a, 2b.

A motor unit within a muscle is made up of fibres of one type only. They are either all slow-twitch fibres or either all fast-twitch fibres. If this unit is contracted for slow exercise, the fibres in it will eventually turn into slow-twitch fibres. If it is contracted for fast movements, the fibres in it will become fast-twitch fibres. This again illustrates that the type of conditioning training done should specifically suit the martial art it is meant to enhance.

Flexibility

Flexibility will affect the range of movement of the muscle around a joint. The greater this range, the more work a muscle can do, provided the angle of pull on the bone is favourable. Another aspect of flexibility is that it reduces resistance to a movement. This means that the muscle will have to do less work to overcome resistance, thereby wasting less energy. This again emphasizes the importance of correct technique.

An awareness of all these factors can become a tool in injury prevention. A knowledge of some basic physiological principles will help eliminate unsafe practices in martial arts classes. These unsafe practices can have a major impact due to the repetitive nature of the techniques performed. Ensuring that the right conditioning takes place so that techniques can be executed in an optimum way will certainly reduce the risk of injury.

Power is determined by all of the above aspects. The muscle has to be able to move a load at speed to make a movement powerful. Mathematically speaking, the faster a heavy load is moved, the more power is required. Strength training should precede training for power. Initially, heavy loads are moved quite slowly. As strength increases and the condition of the muscles and connective tissues

improves, the speed of movement may be increased, turning slow-twitch muscles into fast-twitch muscles.

Preparatory Sessions

Preparatory sessions are vital for anyone working towards teaching or learning a skill or activity that is quite complex. For example, in order to enhance a student's fighting ability for competition in any of the arts that are conducted standing up, an instructor might seek to include plyometric training, in order to enhance mobility and bound. This type of training would be very strenuous on muscles, tendons and bones, and should not be undertaken without adequate strengthening of the muscles and tendons involved. Embarking on such a method of training without the necessary preparation would be likely to lead to serious injury.

Long-term planning and vision is very important. In order to reduce the risk of injury, sessions need to work progressively towards the desired goal. This means, in simple terms, that low-grade sessions should include conditioning work that is of a lower level than the work included in high-grade sessions. The classes should be separated, as the calibre of performance within them is quite different. Like the conditioning work, the technical aspect will also be different. Very often, the need to separate classes is recognized on a technical level, but the conditioning aspect is ignored. The goals set for a class should be hard yet attainable and this cannot be done efficiently if too many skill levels are mixed in the same class. This means that the preparatory session should be considered not only from a physical perspective, but should also account for the mental and technical perspective.

The process of learning skills must be considered when designing classes, and the

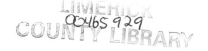

instructor needs to allow for the three stages of learning:

1. *cognitive stage:* this stage is concerned with beginners. Individuals are very much dependent on feedback when learning new skills; they make significant demands on the instructor, as they cannot yet conceptualize what they are doing right and what they are doing wrong. The instructor at this stage should emphasize the nature of the task or technique, rather than the outcome, and should aim to break down techniques into smaller components;
2. *intermediate or associative stage:* at this stage the martial artists can understand more specific instructions and is more efficient and confident. He can interpret his own movements and start correcting them. Techniques should have become more automatic and there should be less thinking about what to do;
3. *autonomous stage:* by this stage, the students do not require a lot of feedback for their skills, absorbing everything easily and interpreting their own movements and correcting them. The instructor will typically use overlearning for such students and comment only on highly specific task components.

Clearly, if the three different skill levels are mixed within the same class, a number of problems may occur. If the sessions are too easy for the individuals who have reached the later stages, those students will lose motivation. If the sessions are too hard, beginners will rush into tasks and techniques, without learning how to do them properly, and may execute them incorrectly. They may also lose motivation because they will repeatedly experience failure. At the lower end of the spectrum, there will be sentiments of disbelief and exhaustion, and at the higher end there is a danger that students will become comfortable and lack concentration. Both instances can result in injuries, as the martial artists' motivation is affected.

Sessions need to be devised properly and planned on a short-term as well as a medium- and long-term basis. Proper insight into this should maintain motivation and prevent injury.

Over-Training

In martial arts, as in any other physical training, it is possible for the individual to over-train. This is most likely if an individual does a lot of auxiliary training to support his martial arts practice. Although training is beneficial to health, too much training can affect health adversely, causing both mental and physical distress for the martial artist.

Over-training or chronic fatigue is most commonly seen in elite performers but it can also occur in keen recreational practitioners who train much more than normal. It will usually present itself as fatigue and under-performance. The martial artist will show a loss of motivation, increased injuries or illnesses, depression, and irritability. If these symptoms remain after a rest period of two weeks, then the martial artist is suffering from over-training syndrome. The occurrence of over-training syndrome is most common when starting to train again after a long break – most martial arts are not seasonal in character, like some sports, but significant breaks do exist in some clubs as they close for holiday periods.

Over-training is the same as being exposed to excess stress. It affects the body in three ways:

1. mechanically: stressing bone tissue, ligaments, muscles and tendons;
2. metabolically: energy-storing molecules needed for muscle contraction are

depleted and stress-related hormones are released. These hormones affect the immune system directly by reducing the immune response, and the individual becomes more susceptible to infection;

3. systemically: the whole system is brought down, the mind is slow and the individual is constantly tired.

Inadequate nutrition can also lead to over-training as insufficient fuel is provided to replace the fuels which are burned during training.

A martial arts instructor or coach must be aware of the symptoms involved in over-training and be able to recognize them. It is vital to allow students to recover after heavy training sessions before exposing them to more hard work. They should be encouraged to get sufficient sleep and eat enough food to replenish their energy stores. If training continues when an individual is suffering from over-training, serious injuries will occur and prolonged illnesses can result.

The time it will take an individual to recover depends on many factors, such as age, genetic make-up, attitude to training, and condition. Recovery from injuries in which bones, tendons or ligaments have been affected will take longer than recovery from injuries that involve only muscles. Energy stores will generally be replenished quite quickly but the mental fatigue may take longer to overcome. If a martial arts instructor suspects that a student may be suffering from over-training, he must send him to seek medical advice.

The Right Attitude

Attitudes Towards Training
The risk of injury can be greatly reduced by participants having the correct attitude towards martial arts training. Once engaged in the activity, each individual should concentrate on what they are doing. Lack of concentration or attention on the part of one person can cause injury to that person, as well as to other parties involved in the class. The psychological fitness of the individual plays an important role in this. Controlling motivation is key to reducing injury risk. The relevant issues can be addressed in a number of ways.

Traditionally, a session of (oriental) martial arts opens and closes with a short meditative period, allowing practitioners to gather their thoughts and focus on the lesson to come, or the activities they have just finished. An instructor should explain to the individual what sort of things he may try to visualize or contemplate during this brief period before engaging in the activity or after finishing the lesson.

Additionally, the warm-up period is used to 'zone in'. It gives the students time to set aside all the other events they have had to manage during the day and to start concentrating on the lesson. This focusing of the mind will ensure that the individual is less likely to be distracted once engaged in the main body of the class. Once the opening meditative sequence and the warm-up have finished, the individual should have his mind on the class and any other thoughts should be in the background. Similarly, the cool-down and the meditative period at the end of the class allow the individual to wind down from focusing on the class and let the mind drift back to normal activities.

When teaching a class, it is good practice for the martial arts instructor to back up and illustrate his instructions. He should tell students not only 'how' to do things, but also 'why' they should be done in the way that has been requested. Students need to be aware of the reasons why they are asked to act in a certain way in their martial arts training. It will give them more understanding and at the same time give them a feeling of control. The instructor should allow students to ask questions and discuss technical approaches. Many martial arts classes do not employ such an open approach to coaching, but it does help the student to develop a level of responsibility towards his training, at the same time encouraging safe practice and correct technique. Students who are treated in this way are able to take part in classes properly and intelligently and to make informed decisions.

When designing classes for a specific purpose, the instructor must ensure that correct and safe techniques are used to work towards the desired outcome of the session. Unsafe practices, which have not been analysed properly, may cause injury and set people back. If an instructor allows unsafe practices to take place, this will encourage students to adopt those practices and possibly repeat them elsewhere. Individuals must be made aware of the right training tools to employ in order to practise techniques safely. Again, this underlines the importance of students fully comprehending why they should do techniques in one way and not another.

During a class, especially during partner-assisted training, it is extremely important not to allow any 'horse play'. Generally speaking, the martial arts culture brings with it a set of defined rules and discipline. Apart from the deeper philosophical aspects of the culture, these rules and discipline can be used to contribute to safety. For example, while partner training the ceremonial bow may be used before and after practice, as a marker for the onset and the finish of a partner set or drill. This is an important point. Sometimes an individual stops concentrating as soon as the instructor gives the command to stop, yet his opponent may already have initiated a technique that he cannot reverse. Both practitioners must remain vigilant until it is clear that no more techniques are being fired, and they have bowed to each other to mark the end of the set.

Goals and Motivation

Another key aspect of the correct attitude during training is the control of motivation. Generally speaking, in martial arts classes, practitioners will be working towards a visible goal, such as a belt grading or a competition. Later on in an individual's martial arts career, however, goals may become less visible. This is also the case if an individual is not interested in competition, or if gradings and tests are not part of the martial art practised.

It is imperative to keep individuals motivated during training, as lack of motivation could lead to a loss of concentration, which could lead to injury. The setting of appropriate goals is critical as it instils confidence. Confident performers are not only higher achievers; they are also more persistent when confronted with failure. An individual's self-confidence is influenced by his own previous success, observation of others succeeding, verbal persuasion, and the positive or negative interpretation of the actual training outcome – in other words, being able or unable to perform a certain technique, combination or pattern.

An open approach within the martial arts class will also help with the setting of goals. The setting of goals will be much more effective if it is done specifically for the individual, when the martial artist has accepted those goals, and when he perceives that the situation lies totally within his control – that is to say, he wants to be in the situation and wants to achieve the set goals.

There should be a minimum influence of other people on targets set. This means that, once the instructor and student have agreed upon a goal, it must be ensured that others cannot sway the student from working towards it. Goals set to help the martial artist work towards a competition, or through a sustained training period, should be organized as a set of multiple short-term goals or milestones. This will provide a great amount of feedback and help sustain self-confidence. This principle can also be used with a whole class. When working with a group of individuals with the same level of skill who are all trying to attain their next medium-term goal (probably to pass their next belt), a series of milestones can be created to get them there. As individuals within the group see other group members reach these milestones, they will be more motivated themselves. When coaching a particular individual or group of individuals towards a competition, more personal goals can be set.

Usually, a martial arts syllabus will give medium- and long-term goals towards which the instructor and class should be working. It is recommended that all members of the class should be familiar with the syllabus, so that they have some understanding of what is to come. Generally speaking, it is the instructor's responsibility to design classes that work towards these goals.

The goals set should be difficult yet achievable. The goals must be at least fifty per cent achievable or the student will experience failure. Trying to meet unrealistic goals may enhance performance in the short term as the individual tries to achieve them, however, the actual goal is unlikely to be achieved. This causes failure to be experienced more often than success, which, in the long run, will ruin the individual's self-confidence and enjoyment. With respect to injuries, hard and unachievable goals are a double-edged knife. An individual who is aiming for goals that are very difficult to achieve may put undue strain on his body,

which could result in injury. Someone who repeatedly fails to achieve his goals will be de-motivated; this can lead to careless practice in class, and subsequently to injury.

Medical Support

A physical check before beginning a martial arts session is very important and the martial artist should be encouraged to tell the instructor about any illness or injury he may have before the session commences. The risk of injury is greatly increased when an instructor or an individual in a class is unaware of any medical conditions or injuries that may be present. The physical check should reduce this particular risk, but it is very limited as a tool, so there are some other guidelines to be aware of.

As when starting any other physical activity, it is advisable for an individual new to martial arts to consult their doctor, especially if they have not been engaged in any other physical activity. Martial arts training comprises many sudden powerful bursts as part of explosive techniques, and requires a lot of stamina, so it is important to ensure that the heart is in a healthy condition and the blood pressure is within acceptable limits. Instructors should always encourage newcomers to undergo a medical check-up.

Although a pre-participation check-up by a doctor is unlikely to detect new issues in a fit, young individual, a simple physical check and interview is still very useful. The doctor should ask about cases in the subject's close family of heart attack before the age of fifty, and collapse, sudden shortness of breath, or palpitations during exercise. He will be able to determine whether conditions such as diabetes, high blood pressure and chest diseases are present. Exercise-induced asthma is another very common complaint that may be detected.

If the instructor is made aware of any

condition the student may have, he will be able to take this into account, and modify or eliminate any exercises that could worsen the situation. Doctors and/or consultants can advise on what exercises to do and which ones to avoid.

The greater an individual's involvement in sporting activity and the higher the level at which it is practised, the more important medical support becomes. Regular checks are vital as the injury risk is increased with a rise in the concentration and volume of an activity; and, as the risk increases, the actual number of injuries sustained will also increase.

A martial arts instructor or coach does not have the same expertise as a medical professional and should not overstep the mark in this respect. It has been known for instructors to abuse their authority over their students and propose a diagnosis for something outside their field. Instructors must know their limits and should always advise the student to seek the help of a trained professional in such cases.

Within these parameters, martial arts instructors need to keep up-to-date with their knowledge of first aid and must be able to administer it if required. In addition, it is strongly recommended that, as well as the instructor, at least one other senior member of the class should be able to administer first aid.

When administering first aid, it is important not to do anything to worsen the situation. First aid should be administered immediately and as a temporary measure. For detailed information on first-aid procedure relating to martial arts injuries, see Chapters 5–10. Anything beyond the scope of first aid must be handled by a medical professional, and, in case of emergency, the instructor must have a fail-safe way of contacting the emergency services immediately.

Environment and Equipment

A Safe Environment

In a typical martial arts class, several pairs of people will be moving around in a defined space. Most of the time, they will be barefoot. The premises where martial arts classes are conducted must meet certain health and safety standards, and a number of key aspects must be considered before choosing a venue. Failure to adhere to the minimum standards can lead to serious injury caused by negligence and lack of vigilance. Most of the aspects listed below will be covered by a common-sense approach, but students and instructors need to be aware of them, as they could all be related to possible injury.

Adequate space Any obstacles within the training area should be assessed and made safe. Radiators and supporting beams may need to be covered. Any objects that protrude into the room must be clearly visible and securely fixed, so that they cannot fall on to anybody, and there is a reduced risk of running into them. Kit bags must also be kept out of the way. The space should be big enough for the particular activity and for the number of people in the class. Be aware of low ceilings and light fixings, especially when training with weapons or executing big throws. Unused equipment should be stored out of the way to avoid congestion.

Ensure that everybody is aware of emergency procedures and exits and that these are easily accessible. The instructor should have a way of contacting the emergency services if they are needed. If the facility does not have a public telephone, the instructor must have a mobile telephone with him.

Light It is important to have sufficient

lighting, which allows the students to see on-coming blows. Insufficient lighting will be a strain on the eyes and can lead to headaches. This in turn will lead to loss of concentration, which will of course increase the risk of injury to the students. Equally, the lights must not dazzle the student as this could also cause problems. Lights should be protected to avoid them from being smashed and causing injury.

Floor surface Most martial arts are done barefoot. Footwear protects the skin of the feet against possible lacerations and friction burns, as well as supporting the ankle joint and absorbing impact with the floor. Wearing no protective footwear therefore poses an additional injury risk, which needs to be reduced as much as possible.

It is necessary to look carefully at the floor to see whether it is sprung, what material it is made of and whether it has any holes, cracks or splinters. For most martial arts, a sprung wooden floor is ideal. However, care must be taken not to let the floor get too slippery as a result of accumulating moisture (*see* the information on ventilation, below). On a more solid surface such as concrete, the risk of injury due to falls or impact is increased. In this case, it is advisable to cover the floor with mats.

Some martial arts require mats all the time – arts that focus on throwing and groundwork should always be done on a matted surface – and the condition of the mats is important. They should not slip apart, creating gaps in which students can get their feet stuck. This will almost certainly lead to ankle injuries. Similarly, the surface material of the mats should have no tears, as feet or toes could get stuck in these holes and lead to nasty injuries.

The floor surface should offer stability but should not have too much grip, which would prevent twisting of the feet. The inability of the foot to pivot with a movement could lead to knee injuries.

Often, facilities are shared with other sportspeople who do wear some kind of footwear. The rules may stipulate that they should wear only indoor shoes, but this is not always the case, and debris, from soil to glass to small stones, may be left on the floor. This can lead to nasty cuts.

Regardless of what kind of material the floor surface is made of, it is crucial that it is clean before the class commences. If there are no staff at the facility to ensure it is clean, the martial arts instructor needs to implement some kind of system, to cover this – perhaps a rota of students to run a mop over the floor before and after each class.

Any blood should be cleaned up off the floor immediately using an antiseptic cleaner, as certain blood-borne diseases can survive for many weeks outside the body. The risk of contamination via small cuts in the feet is therefore great.

Heating The room should have an ambient temperature of 17–18 degrees centigrade. If this temperature cannot be reached, it may be necessary to wear additional clothing in order to maintain a suitable body temperature for safe training. This could become an issue in a martial arts class as practitioners usually wear a traditional uniform and instructors do not make exceptions even under the above circumstances.

If the room is too hot, heat exhaustion will set in, so it is necessary to have adequate ventilation, as well as a supply of drinking water.

Ventilation Ventilation is vital to keep the room at the right temperature, and to maintain a good supply of oxygen. This can be accomplished via air-conditioning machines, extractor fans or even simply opening doors or windows. As long as there is an adequate supply of oxygen, premature fatigue should be avoided. The circulating air will also moderate the temperature, which should prevent any bodies over-heating.

Poor ventilation could cause a film of liquid to form on cold surfaces, including the floor, which will make them slippery. Excess sweat dripping on to the floor will also make it dangerous. Any moisture accumulating on the floor must be mopped up immediately to avoid anybody slipping and injuring himself.

Hygiene Facilities must be kept clean – not just the actual training area, but also the showers, toilets and changing rooms. Infection can occur anywhere and poorly kept facilities will add to the risk. In addition, any equipment used for training must be clean and disinfected when needed.

Protective Equipment

If your martial art or type of training demands extra protective equipment, it must meet the necessary requirements. Mats must be well maintained and fit together properly, so that there are no gaps between them. Other safety equipment includes mitts or gloves, groin guards, chest guards, mouth guards, shin guards, impact shields or focus mitts, helmets, joint supports, and more.

Instructors and students must be aware of the safety demands of a session and no one should engage in an activity that requires protective equipment if that equipment is not available. In most cases, the risk of injury is not due to people not using protective equipment, but to the use of equipment that is no longer, or has never been, adequate for purpose for which it is used. Using faulty equipment can lead to injury of the person wearing or using the equipment, or to injury of the person on whom it is being used. For example, a torn mitt or glove could catch the eye of an opponent or trap an opponent's finger. Similarly, if a helmet used for contact sparring does not fit adequately, terrible injuries could result.

Any practitioners who wear glasses should wear either safety glasses or contact lenses when engaging in sparring activities.

When weapons are used, they need to be intact. Any defect could lead to the weapon, or part of it, being catapulted out of the practitioner's hand and hitting another student.

All equipment should be stored and maintained in a suitable manner. Failure to do this will lead to deterioration of the equipment, which in practice may cause injury to all parties involved. To avoid equipment getting damaged, or being tampered with, it should preferably be locked away.

Clearly, the use and assessment of equipment should be based on common sense. If a piece of equipment, protective or otherwise, is necessary, but it does not meet the standard that is required of it – if it does not fit properly, is damaged, or is not specifically designed for your intended activity – do not use it. If an activity in your martial arts class requires the use of adequate equipment, and adequate equipment is not available, the activity should not be allowed to take place.

3 Principles of Injury Prevention II – Correct Training and Body Maintenance

Correct Movement and Biomechanics

In order for a martial arts instructor to be able to improve his students' movement and execution of techniques, it is imperative to have some basic knowledge of the joint structures in the body. Often, techniques are taught in a way that is damaging to joints because there is a lack of this knowledge. As long as the instructor has a good understanding of the mechanics behind correct movement and technique, the risk of joint injury, whether acute or chronic, will be dramatically reduced.

Structure of Joints

Joints are the places of the body where bones meet. The majority of joints are freely movable – they are said to be *diarthrodial* or *synovial* – and these are the only joints that will be discussed here. They are located in the shoulders, hips, elbows, knees, spine, wrists, ankles, hands and feet. Other classifications of joints, which will not be discussed, are *amphiarthrodial* (allowing slight movement) and *synarthrodial* (allowing no movement).

A synovial joint is bounded by ligaments and has a joint cavity between the bones. This cavity is filled with synovial fluid needed for lubrication, secreted by the synovial membrane. Muscles, which are attached to the bones via tendons, extend across the joint, allowing movement to occur around the joint. Normally, the joint cavity is small, containing only little synovial fluid. An injury, however, can cause extra fluid to be secreted and the joint to swell.

There are six different types of synovial joint, and each type of joint has certain types of movement associated with it. The design of a joint dictates the movements to which it

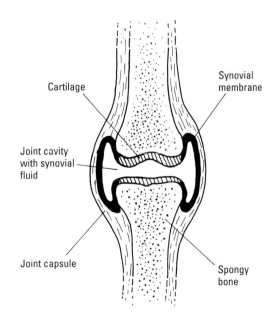

A synovial joint.

Labels on diagram: Cartilage; Synovial membrane; Joint cavity with synovial fluid; Joint capsule; Spongy bone

is suited. It is important to know what these movements are and to have some understanding of which joints are designed to move in which planes.

Gliding joint   Gliding joints include the collarbone, certain joints of the spine, joints in the hands and feet. They are small joints, allowing small gliding movements.

Hinge joint   Hinge joints include the elbow, the knee, the jaw and the ankle. They permit movement in one plane only.

Pivot joint   Pivot joints include the atlantoaxial joint (head movement) and the radioulnar joint (lower arm).

Ellipsoid joint   Ellipsoid joints can be found in the wrists and fingers. They permit movement in two planes at right-angles to each other.

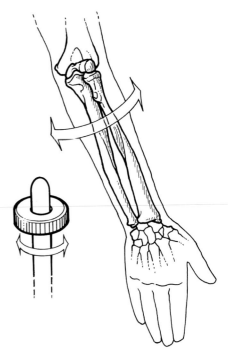

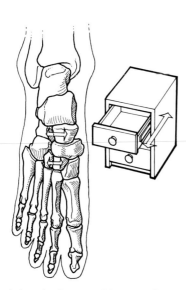

Gliding joints in the tarsal bones of the foot.

Pivot joint: radio-ulnar joint of the forearm.

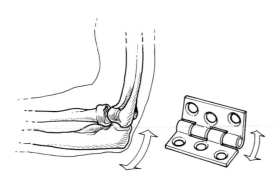

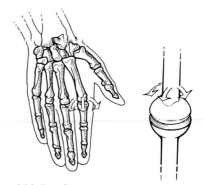

Hinge joint: elbow.

Ellipsoid joint: fingers.

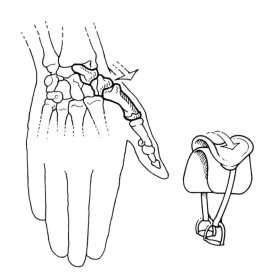

Saddle joint: thumb.

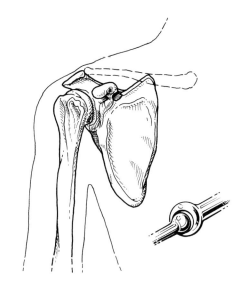

Ball-and-socket joint: shoulder.

Saddle joint One example of a saddle joint is the thumb. Like an ellipsoid joint, it permits movement in two planes at right-angles to each other.

Ball-and-socket joint Ball-and-socket joints include the shoulder and the hip. They are the joints with the widest range of motion.

Movement through Joints

Joint movement is determined by range of motion. Most movement at a joint is of a circular nature, with the bones moving around an axis (joint) in a certain direction. The direction in which they move, and the range of motion of the joint, are determined by several factors. The structure of the bones at, and close to, their articulating ends will influence the range of motion. This means that the shape of the surface of the bones at or near the joint, and the level at which they accept each other will determine the amount of motion the joint can produce. Next, the range of motion is influenced by the joint type. Motion can be limited in a joint due to the impinging of bony structures near or in the joint. A ball-and-socket joint (hip, shoulder) typically allows a wide range of movement in all directions, whereas a hinge joint (knee, elbow) restricts the direction and the range as one bone impinges on another.

The opposite action of muscle groups will also reduce the movement about a joint. As the agonist flexes the joint, the antagonist will produce extension of the joint (*see* page 17, Developing Power). If movement of a joint is made too rapidly into the extreme range of the joint, the antagonist will contract strongly as part of a protective reflex to prevent the joint from being damaged.

The length and the elasticity of the ligaments of the joint are also determining factors. The ligaments assist in limiting joint movement if the muscles fail to contract in a protective manner. The longer and more elastic the ligaments are, the larger the range of motion becomes. Another factor is the elasticity or the ability of the connective tissue of the joint to stretch and return to its original length. This factor can be influenced by physical activity undertaken.

Temperature also influences the range of motion – it has been shown that it is easier to mobilize a joint in a warm environment. With age, it becomes more difficult to mobilize a joint. Generally speaking, women appear to be more flexible than men and therefore have a greater range of motion in their joints.

Joint movements can be described in the following terms:

- *flexion:* a movement that brings two bones closer together, decreasing the angle between them;

- *extension:* a movement that moves two bones away from each other, increasing the angle between them; the opposite of flexion. Hyperextension is extension beyond the normal anatomical position;
- *abduction:* movement of a bone away from a midline;
- *adduction:* a movement of a bone toward a midline;
- *medial rotation:* the turning of a bone on its own axis towards the midline of the body;
- *lateral rotation:* the turning of a bone on its own axis away from the midline of the body.

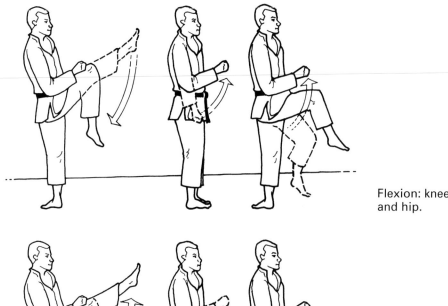

Flexion: knee, elbow and hip.

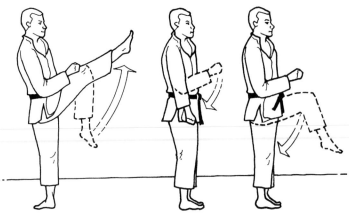

Extension: knee, elbow and hip.

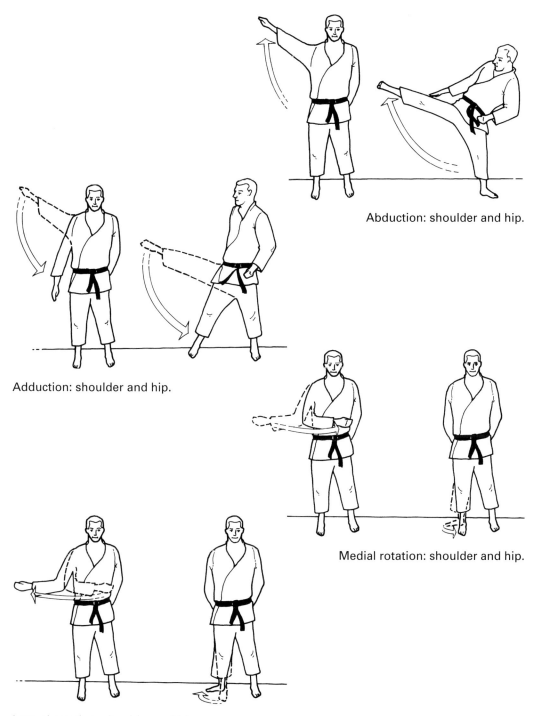

Abduction: shoulder and hip.

Adduction: shoulder and hip.

Medial rotation: shoulder and hip.

Lateral rotation: shoulder and hip.

It is useful to be familiar with each joint and with the movements it allows.

Shoulder The shoulder is a ball-and-socket joint, therefore it is able to move in all directions. Shoulder movements can be enhanced by movement of the scapula (shoulder blade). The shoulder allows the following movements: flexion and extension; abduction and adduction (vertical as well as horizontal); lateral and medial rotation; circumduction (circular movement of the arm).

Elbow The elbow is a hinge joint, therefore it allows movement in one plane only. It allows the following movements: flexion and extension.

Radioulnar joint This joint is a pivot joint. It allows the following movement: rotation (of radius about ulna). This rotation consist of supination (palm faces up) and pronation (palm faces down).

Wrist The wrist is an ellipsoid joint. It allows movement in two planes: up and down; side to side. It allows the following movements: flexion and extension; abduction and adduction (radial flexion and ulnar flexion).

Spine (intervertebral arches) The vertebrae of the spine are made up of gliding joints. They allow sideways movement in two planes as well as rotation. Only a particular section of the spine is involved in the movement; for example, tilting the head backwards does not affect the rest of the spine. The spine allows the following movements: rotation; flexion (bending forwards); hyperextension (bending backwards); lateral flexion (bending to the side).

Hip Very similar to the shoulder, the hip is a ball-and-socket joint. It therefore allows movement in all directions. However, due to the deepness of the socket and tightness of the ligaments, the range of motion is less than that of the shoulder. It allows the following movements: flexion and extension; abduction and adduction (vertical as well as horizontal); lateral and medial rotation; circumduction (circular movement of the leg).

Knee The knee is a hinge joint. Strictly speaking, it therefore allows movement in one plane only. It allows the following movements: flexion and extension. In the flexed position the knee may also allow a *limited* amount of rotation, abduction and adduction. The key word here is 'limited'. In many martial arts the twisting or pushing inwards of the knee when the majority of the body weight rests on the joint leads to chronic injuries. Examples might include failing to rotate the standing leg in kicking so that the knee takes the strain of the required rotation, and pushing the knee inwards when standing in a deep stance, thereby moving the joint out of the natural alignment of the upper and lower leg.

Ankle The ankle is a hinge joint and therefore moves in one plane only. It allows the following movements: plantar flexion (extension); dorsiflexion (flexion); limited rotation.

Intertarsal joint This joint is responsible for the sideways movement of the foot at the base of the ankle. It is a gliding joint allowing the knife-edge of the foot to be pushed out or upwards. It allows the following movements: inversion (foot blade out and down); eversion (lifting the blade of the foot up).

Joint movements are caused by forces that work on the levers around a fulcrum. In the body, the bones are the levers, and the joint is the fulcrum. Forces are used either to facilitate or prevent movement around a joint. The forces that cause this movement around a joint are usually the result of muscle contractions or gravity, although extrinsic forces such as a person pulling or pushing can also make a joint move. Whether or not movement in a joint occurs depends on whether the amount of force used to initiate the movement overcomes the sum of the forces generated by friction and the resistance generated by forces opposing the movement.

Muscle contractions can also be used to resist the movement of a joint (*see* page 17, Developing Power). A muscle can contract to avoid an external force attempting to move a joint, such as another person manipulating the joint or the joint being moved by gravity (for example, in lifting weights).

In order to prevent chronic or even acute injuries to joints, either of which will take a long time to heal, it is vital to be very vigilant and ensure that correct motion through the joint is encouraged. Prolonged bad technique will lead to serious injury of a joint. The techniques taught in a martial arts class must therefore be critically analysed for their movement components and a sound approach to teaching those techniques must be synthesized in order to avoid incorrect movement.

It is necessary to work on the enhancement of the range of motion of joints as required in the specific martial art being practised. This means improving the elasticity of the connective tissue and tendons of the joint. This, together with the improvement of flexibility of the muscles, will increase the agility of the student. Time must be allowed for the adaptation to take place. Connective tissue (ligaments and tendons) takes longer to adjust to new loads than muscles do, and a slow progression is therefore recommended.

For the martial artist there is a conflict of interest here. Generally, martial artists require a lot of flexibility in their joints, but a joint that allows a bigger range of motion may also be less stable. Instructors must give special attention to strengthening the muscles around a joint. Care must be taken to balance the increase in flexibility of the joint with the required strength of muscle around that joint in order to provide enough stability. This will help to support the joint through movements that require it to extend to the extremes of its range. The muscles must be able to provide the protective reflex to stop excessive movement. Many martial arts techniques are of an explosive nature. Not only must the muscles be able to fire off these techniques, but they must also be able to stop them. Proper conditioning of the muscles concerned will reduce the risk of injury to joint structures, which can take a long time to heal. If the muscle strength does not compensate for the increased range of motion and resultant decrease in stability in the joint, injuries to connective tissue, such as sprains and dislocations of the joints, will become more likely.

Warming Up

Reasons for a Warm-Up

Light endurance activities and stretching must be included before and after a workout. A martial arts class, like most other activity classes, will dynamically work large-muscle groups at high intensity and long enough to put sufficient stress on the cardio-respiratory system. Each class should be working towards a specific goal. Sometimes the contents of the class will be of a more technical nature; sometimes the exercises will be of a more fitness-enhancing nature. In either case, the warm-up should add to the potential of the body in the main part of the class, not detract from it.

A warm-up is a preparatory set of exercises designed to enable the body to do the work in the main session. Warming up should not be tiring or difficult, but should involve a set of steadily increasing aerobic, callisthenic exercises, moving the body into an optimum state to do the main exercises of the martial arts session. Aerobic metabolism supplies energy by burning carbohydrates and fatty acids using oxygen. Callisthenic exercises are done without equipment and are performed for flexibility and muscular development.

Any hard exercise at this stage will lead to partial exhaustion of certain muscle groups, which could lead to injury when the muscles are made to work at full capacity in the main part of the class. All too often, the warm-up is too demanding for the class and some of the major muscle groups have been fatigued before the technical martial arts practice begins. It is bad practice to make students do a huge amount of press-ups and sit-ups as part of their warm-up, although this is done in many dojos. Physical conditioning – that is to say, the improvement of strength – should not be part of the warm-up. Indeed, a separate section of the class should be devoted specifically to this subject.

A useful guideline for a warm-up is to include exercises similar to those that will be done in the main section of the class, but to do them at a lower intensity. The muscles that will be utilized in the main part of the class should be stretched, along with the muscles of the abdominal area and lower back, which are involved in all moves to stabilize the body. These particular muscles must be thoroughly warmed up if they are not to be damaged when executing martial arts techniques, which are often explosive.

Experience shows that most practitioners of the 'upright' arts, such as karate, taekwondo, kung-fu and kick-boxing, employ some form of aerobic exercise at the beginning of their sessions. However, in 'sit-down' or grappling arts, such as judo and ju-jitsu, this is not always the case. Before these activities, the joints are usually statically stretched, some dynamic stretching drills are done, and then some callisthenic exercise in the form of forward and backward rolling and break-falling follows the stretching. However, it is often the case that nothing is done to optimize the state of the body and prepare it for exercise. This means that techniques such as throws could easily cause injury to the person executing the throw as well as to the person being thrown.

Effects of the Warm-Up

The first effect of a warm-up is the elevation of body temperature. This will result in the following processes. Enzyme activity will be enhanced, which in turn increases metabolism in the muscles. This means that the fuel needed to create the necessary energy for exercising becomes available more easily. Blood flow and oxygen delivery to the muscles will be increased. This again ensures a steady supply of blood-borne fuel – carbohydrates and fatty acids – to the muscles, and the oxygen required to burn it.

Contraction and reflex times in the muscles will be improved and the muscles will be more pliable. A rapid increase in blood pressure will be prevented. Blood flow to the heart will be increased, which reduces any risk to the heart created by the onset of sudden abrupt exercise.

A good warm-up will lessen the likelihood of injury, particularly in high-power tasks, and it will provide a period of psychological preparation associated with increased arousal and readiness.

Contents of a Warm-Up

A warm-up should include the following basic parts:

- physical check;
- gentle joint articulation;
- aerobic warm-up.

A physical check is important to make sure that you have no injuries before starting a session. It will not always be obvious that certain structures of the body might have been damaged due to activities before the session. Small injuries can sneak in undetected, particularly in the martial artist who trains several times a week, and these could develop into worse injuries that may prevent further training or competing.

Before the start of any class, the martial arts coach or instructor must insist that students let him know about any injury or illness they may have. This way, the instructor can adjust or eliminate exercises as necessary in order not to aggravate an existing injury, or cause a new one.

Joint structures (wrists, ankles, neck, hips, knees, shoulders) should be articulated without exerting any force and at slow speed, making sure that possible pains are not masked. Movements must be isolated so that pains and strains can be detected and located.

The aerobic warm-up then focuses on raising body temperature and heart rate. It should not be tiring; it is simply preparing the body for exercise. Students should work up a light sweat.

The warm-up should have a general part and a specific part. The general part involves drills that can be done by anybody. The specific part uses techniques that relate to a particular martial art or sport. All relevant muscle groups must be warmed up and any set of exercises may be constructed in order to accomplish this. These exercises can mimic the techniques of the particular martial art, as long as they do not put too much structural strain on the body before it has been thoroughly warmed up.

Below is an example of the sequence of movements and exercises that could be involved in the physical check and gentle joint articulation part of a warm-up.

1. Stand comfortably with feet shoulder-width apart; gently turn the head from side to side; gently raise and lower the head; gently tilt the head from side to side.
2. Make small shoulder rotations in both

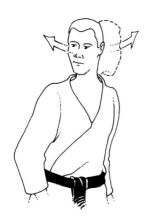 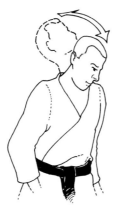 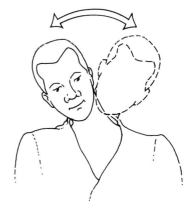

Turn the head side to side.　　Raise and lower the head.　　Tilt the head side to side.

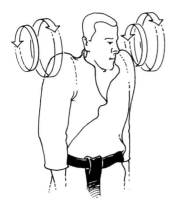

Small shoulder rotations.

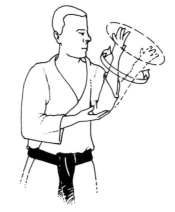

Movement about the elbow.

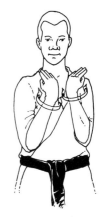

Wrist rotations.

directions; continue with gentle movement about the elbow; make slow wrist rotations in both directions.

3. Make small and gentle rotations of the waist in both directions, paying attention to the lower back; gently push the hips forward and backwards.

4. Rotate the knees in both directions, making sure the feet stay flat on the floor.

5. Slowly articulate both ankles by rotating the foot, resting on the ball of the foot with the ankle raised off the floor. Make small circles in both directions.

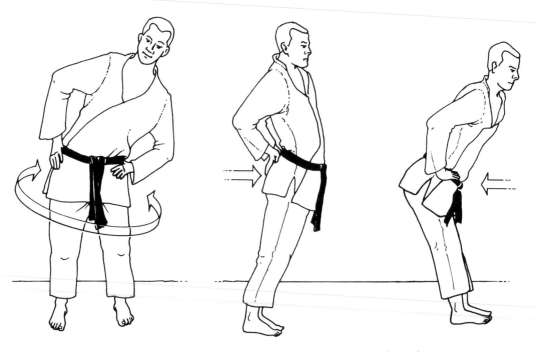

Rotation of the waist.

Push the hips forwards and backwards.

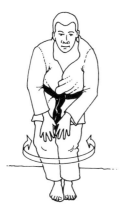

Rotation of the knees.

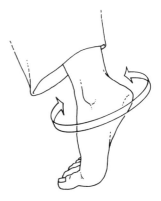

Articulation of both ankles.

For the aerobic section of the warm-up, try the sequence below.

1. Gentle bouncing up and down or jogging on the spot to raise the level of circulation; progress into Jumping Jacks, to raise the circulation in legs and arms; vary the Jumping Jacks by rotating the body to alternate sides while opening legs and arms.
2. Execute striking techniques while bouncing in a straddle stance.

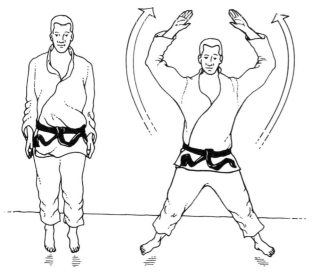

Jumping Jacks.

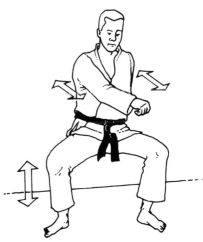

Striking while bouncing in a straddle stance.

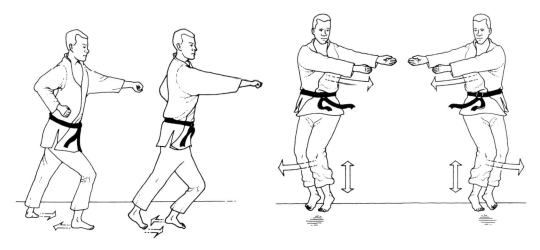

Stride jumps with reverse punches.

Hip twists.

3. Do alternate stride jumps while reverse
   punching on stance changes.
4. Do hip twists while bouncing (as in
   slalom skiing) for warming up the lower
   back and trunk.
5. Step out on alternate sides in a front
   stance executing a striking technique,
   then pull back to starting position.
6. Jog on the spot, alternating heels up/

knees up, putting emphasis on
quadriceps and hamstrings, to
prepare for knee raises and gentle
front kicking while bouncing. This
will warm up gluteus muscles, hip
flexors and extensor, hamstrings and
quadriceps.
7. Do a number of squat thrusts and
   burpees.

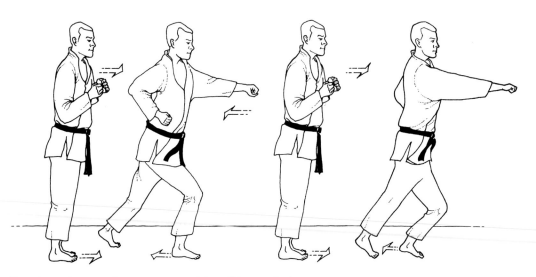

Step into alternate front stances with striking techniques.

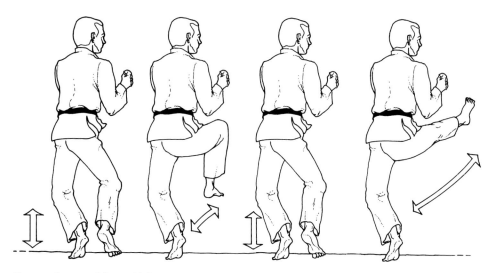

Knee raises and front kicks.

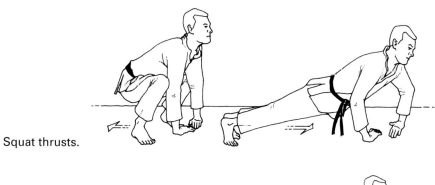

Squat thrusts.

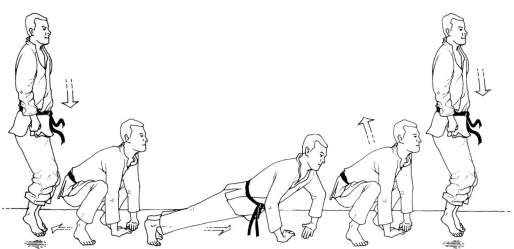

Burpees.

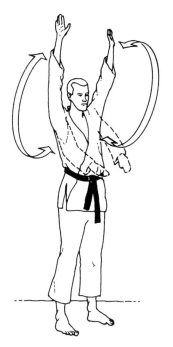

Arm and shoulder rotations.

8. Make arm rotations/shoulder rotations in both directions.

This part of the warm-up can be concluded by some light callisthenics. At this final stage, a number of light strengthening exercises such as press-ups and sit-ups can be included, but they should not fatigue the martial artist and diminish his capacity to do the remainder of the session. The warm-up for a typical one- to two-hour martial arts class should last for fifteen to twenty or thirty minutes. Classes that last longer should allow for breaks, after which a new, shorter warm-up should take place.

The initial section of the main part of the session ought to be a form of formal activity, which will complement the warm-up. It consists of exercises specific to the martial art you practise. These exercises would typically be techniques that occur often within the normal activities of your art.

Stretching

Once the body has been thoroughly warmed up, gentle stretching of the major muscle groups can take place. Depending on the particular martial art practised or the content of the lesson, it might be relevant to spend more time on certain muscle groups.

Although recent research suggests that stretching as part of a warm-up is not always beneficial, in our experience stretching as part of a warm-up in martial arts, followed by some specific techniques relevant to the art, is very important in order to ensure adequate mobilization of the joints.

The stretching routine must not allow the body to cool down again and the instructor should ensure that stretching is interspersed with light activity to keep the circulation up. Another way of keeping the body working while stretching is by including isometric exercises – exercises that keep the working muscles at the same length (*see* page 17, Developing Power: strength, speed and flexibility). For example, you could assume a straddle stance while stretching the arms and upper body. Another idea may be to intersperse static stretches with dynamic ones.

The amount of time a stretch is held should be long enough for the inverse stretch reflex to occur, but not so long that the body temperature drops again. A muscle's initial reaction to being stretched is actually to shorten and resist the stretch. After a certain period of time, processes occur that allow the muscle to relax and lengthen with the stretch.

Stretches should be held initially for six to ten seconds, with the general aim of increasing the time to thirty seconds. The martial artist should stretch gently to the point just before pain sensation, whilst relaxing, and then release slowly from the stretch. In a stretching routine, three or four sets of each exercise, which are each held for thirty seconds, should be performed.

Static Stretches

Static stretches should be performed without jerking. This type of stretch is done correctly by putting the antagonistic muscle (*see* page 17, Developing Power: strength, speed and flexibility) in its most lengthened position and holding it there. The seated hamstring stretch is one example of this type of stretch:

1. sit with both legs extended together in front;
2. gently lower the chest towards the knees and attempt to reach the toes;
3. reaching as far as possible, hold the stretch.

Dynamic Stretches

Dynamic or ballistic stretching uses repetitive contractions of the agonistic muscle (a muscle that is the prime mover in a contraction) to give quick stretches of the antagonistic muscle (a muscle that causes movement at a joint in a direction opposite to that of its agonist, *see* page 17, Developing Power: strength, speed and flexibility). A series of pulls on the resistant muscle is used to increase the range of movement about a joint. A distinction is made between 'continuous force movement' and 'ballistic force movement'. In a continuous force movement, the muscle tension is almost maximal throughout the movement. In a ballistic force movement, the body part is at first moved by a fast, brief contraction of the agonistic muscle, but the muscle force is then reduced and the action continues due to the momentum generated. The speed of movement gradually decreases due to the resistance of the antagonistic muscle, resistance in the joint and external resistance such as gravity.

Because of the short repetitive stretch burst, the inverse stretch reflex is not employed, which means that the muscle is continually resisting the stretch. In martial arts, there are many movements that constitute a dynamic or ballistic stretch. Kicking and punching are perfect examples.

When doing this type of stretching, care must be taken as to the degree to which the muscle and connective tissue are stretched. The action should always take place within the limits of the martial artist's dynamic flexibility. Any bursts that push beyond that dynamic flexibility will cause injuries to the tissues being stretched. There should be no over-stretching and static stretching is vital, to provide a 'buffer zone' in the muscle and connective tissues to allow for those martial arts techniques that are of a ballistic nature.

Stretching Routines

A useful guideline for a stretching routine is to work your way either up or down the body, stretching each muscle group as you get to it. As an instructor, it is important to develop a stretching routine that your students can easily remember and repeat at each session.

In stretching, as in any physiological exercise, bad technique can lead to injuries. Repetition of bad technique on a regular basis will certainly lead to bad habits and symptoms of chronic injury.

It is important to maintain the correct body position when stretching, in order to reduce strain on the neck and the lower back. It is particularly important to maintain the correct alignment of the lower back, head, shoulders and legs. Often, too much strain is put on the upper and lower spine by martial artists arching the spine when trying to increase a stretch.

There are a number of things to observe during stretching to avoid injury:

- make sure that the spine is in line, as this reduces the stress on it. Even when bending forward to enhance a stretch, the spine should be kept as straight as possible;
- keep the head up, looking ahead rather than at the floor. This will reduce stress on the neck and back;
- when doing stretches lying on your back, raise the shoulders and upper back off the floor, as this will reduce stress on the lower back;
- always start by doing preparatory stretching in the warm-up. There should be a clear distinction between the type of stretching done as part of a warm-up or cool-down and that done for flexibility training. The aim of stretching in a warm-up and cool-down is to stretch to the current limitations of the body. Developmental stretching (to improve flexibility) is aimed at improving on the present range of movement and should be done at a later stage in a separate period of the main session.

The following example routine can be done as part of a warm-up. The stretches follow the 'top to bottom' approach, starting with the muscles at the top of the body and working downwards. The structure of a stretching routine will vary depending on the content of the lesson or the emphasis of the martial art you practise.

1. Lateral neck stretch: stand up straight and tilt the head to the side, stretching the muscles on the side of the neck. The stretch may be enhanced by placing the hand on top of the head and gently pulling the head to the side. Repeat on the other side.

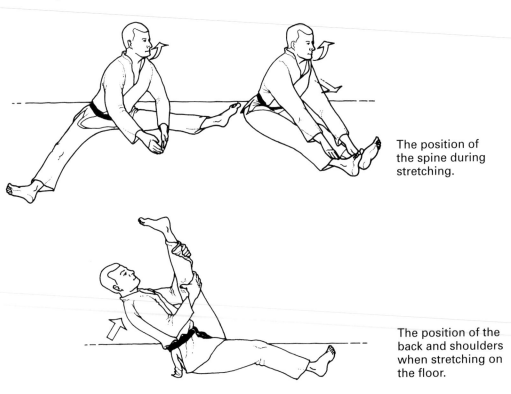

The position of the spine during stretching.

The position of the back and shoulders when stretching on the floor.

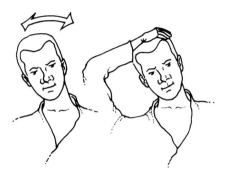

Lateral neck stretch.

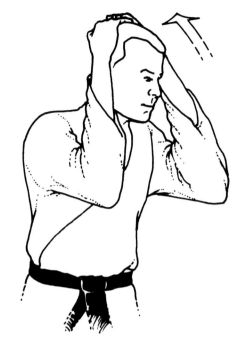

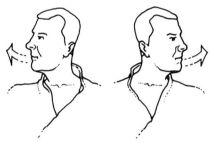

Rotation neck stretch.

Posterior neck stretch.

2. Rotation neck stretch: stand up straight and turn the head as far as possible to one side and hold; repeat on the other side.
3. Posterior neck stretch: stand up straight and lower the chin and clasp both hands on the top of the head. Ensure the back is

not arched when doing this. Keep the head in its current position but press back into the hands.
4. Partial head rotation: stand up straight and drop the chin to the chest. Continue to rotate the head in a circular motion. When the head comes up at the side to

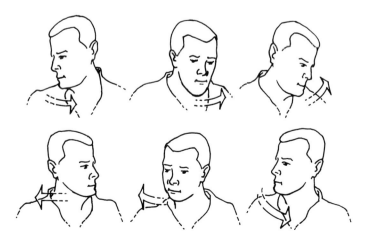

Partial head rotation.

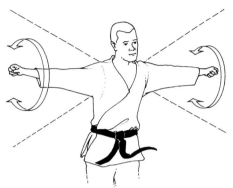

Shoulder rotation.

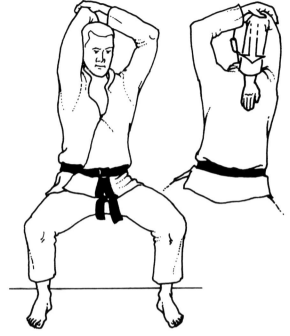

Shoulder stretch.

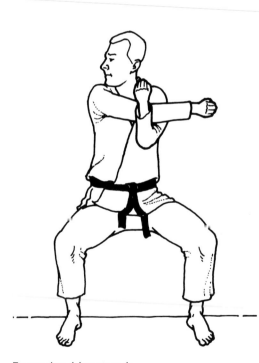

Front shoulder stretch.

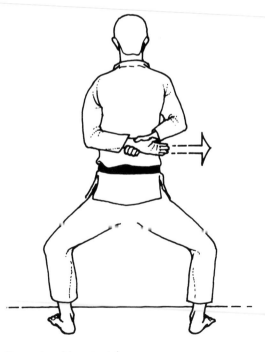

Rear shoulder stretch.

its normal level, gently turn it across to the other side without letting it tilt backwards (this would put undue pressure on the neck). Once on the other side, drop the chin and continue the circular motion.

5. Shoulder rotation: in a standing position, circle the shoulders in both directions, slowly increasing the radius of the circle.

6. Shoulder stretch: raise one elbow and place the hand behind the neck. With the other hand, grab and pull the raised elbow towards the centre line. (This can be done while in a straddle stance, to keep the muscles in the legs working and the body temperature up.)

7. Front shoulder stretch: straighten one arm in front of the chest and use the other arm to pull it in towards the chest. Turn the head towards the shoulder that is being stretched. Keep the straddle stance.

8. Rear shoulder stretch: pass your arm around your back, grab on to your wrist with the other hand and pull. Maintain the straddle stance.

9. Shoulder and chest stretch: clasp hands behind your back and, pressing the

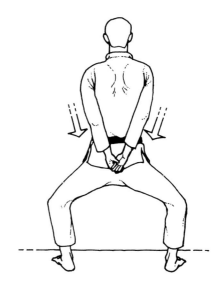

Shoulder and chest stretch.

shoulder blades together, pull down. Keep the straddle stance and pull the stomach in so that the back is not arched.

10. Opening and closing the chest: stand up straight. Cross your arms in front of you and then open up, stretching them out to the side. Repeat this several times, each time changing the arm that goes on top.

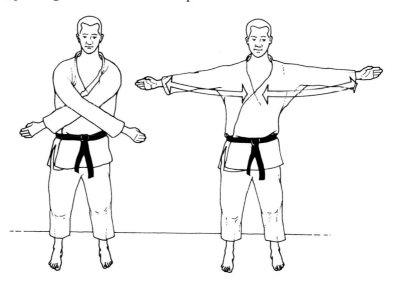

Opening and closing the chest.

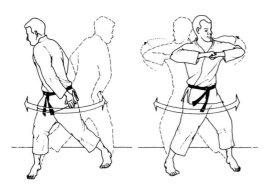
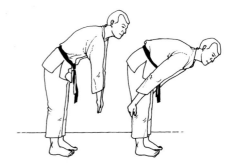

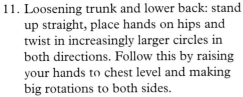

Loosening trunk and lower back.

Hamstring and lower back stretch.

11. Loosening trunk and lower back: stand up straight, place hands on hips and twist in increasingly larger circles in both directions. Follow this by raising your hands to chest level and making big rotations to both sides.

12. Hamstring and lower back stretch: stand up straight. Keeping the feet shoulder-width apart, slowly lower the chest towards the knees. Keep looking forward and keep the chin up. The hands can be placed behind the calves. To increase the stretch, repeat with the feet closer together.

13. Hip flexor stretch: step forward into a front stance and lower the knee of the back leg towards the floor. Keeping the back straight, push the hips forward

and squeeze the buttocks. Repeat on the other side.

14. Inner thigh and hamstring stretch: from the front stance position straighten the back leg, ensuring the back heel remains on the floor. Bring the front knee above the front toes and keep the back straight. After holding this for a while, place both hands on the floor on the inside of the front foot, making sure the chin is kept up to avoid strain on the back. Attempting to keep your hands in that position, straighten the front leg and lower the chest towards the knee. Once again, keep the head up. Repeat this a number of times before changing to the other leg.

15. Straddle stretch: assuming a straddle

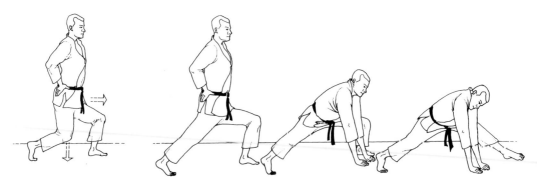

Hip flexor stretch.   Inner thigh and hamstring stretch.

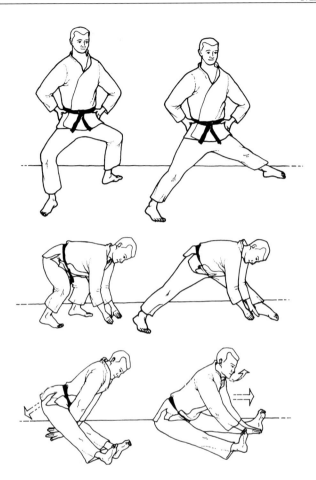

Straddle stretch.

stance, straighten and bend the legs a few
times, keeping the back straight. Then
bend the legs again, place the hands on
the floor in front, and straighten the legs.
Lower the chest to the centre, then lower
it towards each leg. Place the hands
between the legs and behind the line of
the heels and bring the weight on to the
hands, pointing the toes upwards. Sit
down gently from this position and then
repeat the above stretches in the seated
position.

16. Groin stretch: sit down on the floor,
grasp your ankles and pull them in
towards the groin. Use the elbows to
apply downward pressure to the knees.

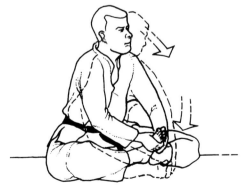

Groin stretch.

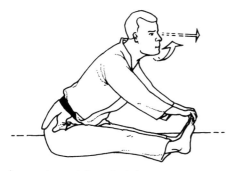

Lower hamstring stretch.

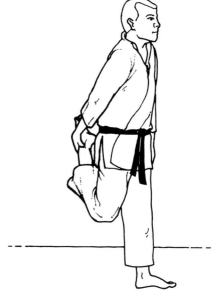

17. Lower hamstring stretch: sit down on the floor, straighten the legs in front and keep the feet together. Reach forward with the hands and grab the ankles or toes. Keep the chin up and look forward, not down.

18. Front thigh stretch: stand up straight. Grab the ankle of your foot and pull the heel up to the buttocks, keeping the knees together and squeezing the hips forward. Repeat on the other leg.

19. Calf and Achilles tendon stretch: stand up straight and slightly bend one leg. Place the heel of the other leg in front, keeping the leg straight. Rest your hands

Front thigh stretch.

on the thigh of the bent supporting leg and press the chest towards the straight leg. To increase the stretch, grasp the raised foot. Keep the chin up and keep looking forward. Repeat on the other leg.

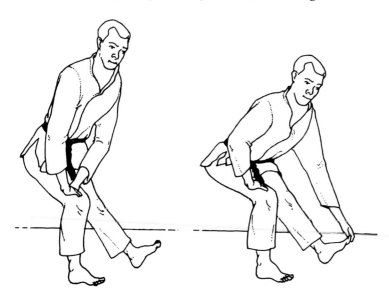

Calf and Achilles
tendon stretch.

20. Knee rotations: stand up straight. Keep the feet together and slightly bend both knees. Place the hands on the knees and gently rotate them in both directions, keeping the feet flat on the floor.

21. Forward leg swings: assume a comfortable front stance and gently swing the back leg forwards and bring it back to its starting position. Repeat on the other side.

22. Backward leg swings: assume a comfortable front stance and gently swing the front leg backwards and bring it back to its starting position. Repeat on the other side.

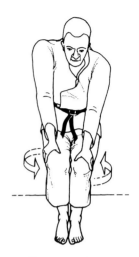

Knee rotations.

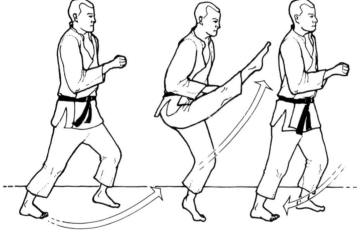

Forward leg swings.

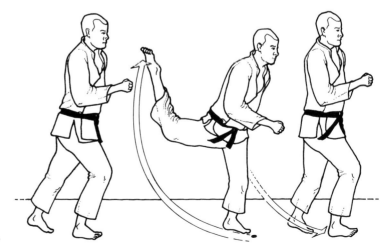

Backward leg swings.

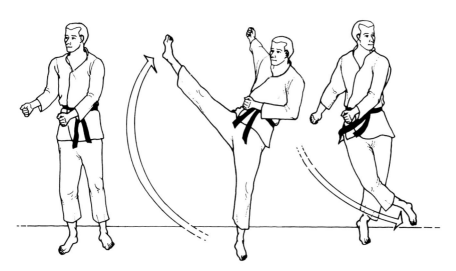

Sideways leg swings.

23. Sideways leg swings: stand with feet shoulder-width apart. Swing one leg away from the body, pointing the foot upwards. Swing the leg across the body, pointing the toes in the direction of the swing. Repeat on the other leg.

Cooling Down

In essence, the cool-down has the opposite purpose of the warm-up. Using exercises similar to those used in the warm-up, the aim is to bring the body back from an active state to a relaxed state. The cool-down will ensure that any residual waste products, such as lactic acid, are removed from the muscles and the blood. This will avoid aches and potential muscle fatigue when starting the next bout of exercise. Remember: starting a session when fatigued can lead to injury.

The cool-down should take five to fifteen minutes. Like the warm-up, it will involve light aerobic exercises, mirroring the exercises done in the main part of the class. It should also include stretching of the muscles that have been worked during the session. The stretches should be held for thirty seconds, although at this stage the duration may be increased in order to achieve greater flexibility.

Many of the techniques in martial arts involve dynamic or ballistic stretching of the muscle, which can cause muscle soreness later. Ten minutes of static stretching after a work-out can prevent this soreness to a significant degree. It must therefore form a part of the cool-down after a martial arts class.

To conclude, a warm shower is recommended as well as a sufficient period of rest before starting the next bout of exercise. Proper fluid replacement is also crucial.

Maintaining the Body

Nutrition

The term 'nutrition' refers to chemicals which are absorbed into the body's systems for use as an energy source and to agents that keep the body healthy. Inadequate nutrition will lead to certain parts of the body being more susceptible to injury. It is therefore crucial to have some understanding of the basics of correct nutrition.

Correct nutrition will be composed of

adequate amounts of the following chemicals:

- carbohydrates;
- fats;
- proteins;
- vitamins;
- minerals, electrolytes and trace elements;
- fibre;
- water.

Of course, the term 'adequate amount' is relative to each individual and also relative to the amount of physical work done. People involved in any sport need to have an understanding of what nutrients they require in their diet to maintain their health, to enable them to perform and to prevent or limit injury or illness. Moreover, if an individual does become injured or ill, the right diet will speed up the recovery process. For individuals attending several martial arts classes a week, it is even more important to have a healthy body that is less prone to injury, and has the ability to recover quickly if injured.

Of the above nutrients, carbohydrates, fats and proteins play a role in energy provision. The other chemicals cannot provide the body with energy. The energy in food is measured in (kilo) calories or in (kilo) Joules. The energy density of nutrients differs significantly. Fats have by far the most energy (thirty-seven kilo Joules per gram), followed by carbohydrates (seventeen kilo Joules per gram) and proteins (sixteen kilo Joules per gram).

Carbohydrates

Simply put, carbohydrates are made up of basic units or monosaccharides. The most common one is glucose. Two basic units can be linked together to form disaccharides – what we consider as sugar. Longer chains of monosaccharides, such as starch, are called polysaccharides.

Carbohydrates are essential for maintaining the body's energy stores, and can be stored in the form of glycogen in muscle tissue and in the liver. Excess glucose that cannot be stored as glycogen will be converted into fat, which is very readily stored in tissue all over the body.

Carbohydrates are usually divided into simple carbohydrates and complex carbohydrates. The simple carbohydrates, such as sugar, are the most readily usable for exercise. Complex carbohydrates, such as starch, must be broken down into simple carbohydrates before they can provide energy, in a process that occurs over a period of time. As complex carbohydrates also contain vitamins and minerals, it is recommended to take on this type of carbohydrate, because this ensures the provision of such nutrients. Individuals who do a lot of physical work or exercise can consume simple carbohydrates without too great a risk of weight gain.

Carbohydrates are the energy source used during the onset of any exercise and the only source of energy during high-intensity exercise. They are also needed for the efficient digestion of fat. Carbohydrates will be used to stack the glycogen stores that come into play in an explosive martial arts technique, and other techniques that require high-level aerobic activity.

Fats

The structure of a fat molecule consists of long tails and a head. The tails are chains of fatty acids and the head is a glycerol group. Fats can be divided into three groups: saturated fats, mono-unsaturated fats and polyunsaturated fats. They are required as part of a healthy diet, although only in small amounts. The body can build its own fatty acids from components it has stored, but it cannot synthesize certain fatty acids. These must be absorbed as part of the diet.

Fats are important nutrients. They

provide energy as well as a means of synthesizing many essential components and tissues that are vital to the functioning of the body. Certain fatty acids are needed to repair and maintain tissues such as tendons and ligaments. Fats help in the uptake of vitamins A, D, E and K. Fats are the prime energy source during prolonged low-level exercise. A certain percentage of body fat is required for the martial artist to take part in prolonged aerobic training.

Proteins

Proteins are large molecules made up of various amino acids. Most amino acids can be constructed by the body by breaking down proteins and amino acids and putting them together again. As with fats, however, there are certain essential amino acids that the body cannot make; these need to be provided by the diet.

Amino acids are required for structural components of the body (muscle), haemoglobin (blood), hormones and enzymes, brain, heart, organs and skin. They are not a preferred source of energy and can only contribute a maximum of ten per cent to energy provision during exercise. Carbohydrates and fats are the primary fuels during exercise.

There is a general misconception that lots of protein needs to be consumed in order to produce more muscle tissue. In fact, this is not the case. Only an adequate amount of protein is required in the diet, to supply essential amino acids, as the body will only use what it needs at a given moment to construct, repair or replenish tissue. (In martial arts, due to the impact experienced in training, this is very important.) Any excess protein will leave the body.

As long as enough carbohydrates are taken in, the body will synthesize the required muscle protein in the muscle tissue using glycogen. Only individuals under-

taking extreme heavy resistance training, or bodybuilding, may need to increase their protein intake.

Vitamins

'Vitamin' is a short term for 'vital amine'. Vitamins are compounds needed to perform specific tasks within the body such as growth and development. They facilitate key processes within the body. Certain vitamins help reduce harmful free oxygen radicals, which can be the cause of many diseases. Generally, obvious signs of vitamin deficiency are rare in the developed world, but low vitamin levels may impair sports performance or recovery from injury or illness.

Vitamins are either water- or fat-soluble. The water-soluble vitamins include the vitamin B complexes and vitamin C. The fat-soluble vitamins include vitamin A, D, E and K.

Some of the functions of certain vitamins are particularly relevant in this context. Vitamin A is mainly associated with good eyesight and skin. It is also involved in maintaining and repairing connective tissue such as tendons and ligaments. Several vitamin B compounds are involved in the metabolism of energy molecules and the creation of red blood cells. Vitamin B_1 is involved in breaking down sugars to provide energy in muscles. Vitamin B_2 also helps with the breakdown of carbohydrates, but its main function is to help turn fats and proteins into carbohydrates, which can then be used to provide energy in exercise. A lack of this vitamin will reduce performance. Vitamin B_3 is necessary for the breakdown of glucose into energy. Vitamin B_6 aids in building proteins from amino acids and is important for building muscle. Vitamin B_{12} is required for building up red blood cells, which is important to ensure that the blood's capacity to transport the oxygen needed for the burning of fuel is maintained. All together, it is very obvious why a martial artist requires an adequate supply of the vitamin B complex. It is essential to ensure that energy-storing molecules can be burned, oxygen can be provided and muscle tissue can be built.

Vitamin C is essential in the production of collagen, which is found in connective tissue (tendons and ligaments) and bones. It is also important for any healing process and helps the body absorb iron. Vitamin E acts as an anti-oxidant by keeping vitamins A and C and fatty acids from being destroyed in the blood. Vitamins C and E are therefore very important for exercise and avoiding and/or recovering from injury. Vitamin K is required for the blood-clotting process, which is essential to stop bleeding.

Minerals, electrolytes and trace elements
These are chemicals that are required by the body in small amounts. Largely, they will be needed for mechanisms involved in the nervous system. Some are also needed for correct functioning of glands and formation of bone, teeth, enzymes, and so on. Certain compounds are also required for parts of energy metabolism. For example, iron is important, as it is needed to form haemoglobin for red blood cells to transport oxygen to exercising muscles.

Fibre
Fibre is a non-digestible carbohydrate, which is not absorbed by the body. It is essential to ensure proper functioning of the intestines as food masses pass through them.

Energy Provision in Martial Arts Exercise
It is not possible to say exactly how much energy a martial artist needs for a typical day, as this will vary from individual to individual. If more energy is consumed than is needed, the excess will be stored as fat and the body weight will increase. If insufficient energy is consumed, the body will use its energy stores to meet the demands of exercise and the body weight will reduce. Energy stored in the body should be released at an adequate rate to meet the body's demand for energy, particularly during exercise.

Carbohydrates and fats are the major contributors in energy provision during exercise. Protein can only account for up to ten per cent of the energy provided. A martial arts class will consist of a spectrum of aerobic and anaerobic exercise. During low-intensity aerobic exercise, the body will use a mixture of carbohydrates and fats to provide the required energy. As the intensity increases, so does the proportion of carbohydrates used to meet the energy demand. During high-intensity anaerobic work, carbohydrate is the only energy source.

During long events or classes (those lasting longer than sixty minutes), the body's stored carbohydrate will become the limiting factor for performance levels. Although even the slimmest athlete carries a large fat storage, it is the ability to store carbohydrates that becomes important in prolonged activities. Through training, the body's ability to store carbohydrates in the form of glycogen is increased. Another effect of training is that the body will use a higher percentage of fat, thus saving the important glycogen in order to prolong performance.

A low carbohydrate intake coupled with hard training will lead to low glycogen levels in the muscles. This will bring on fatigue more easily and performance will be reduced. These two aspects can lead to injuries, as technique and its execution may be affected. It is important for a martial arts instructor or coach to realize that hard training days should therefore be followed by rest days, in order for muscle glycogen to be replenished.

Adequate nutrition is vital for the prevention of and recovery from injuries. It will ensure that tissues are well stocked with the correct chemicals so that exhaustion is less likely. The body's tissues should be in good shape if all the correct compounds form part of the diet; structural weaknesses will be avoided, thereby reducing the risk of injuries. If injuries do occur, recovery will be hastened if the correct nutrition is provided. If all the necessary chemicals are readily available, the body will be able to repair more easily. Due to the nature of the martial arts, the ability of tissue to repair readily is very important.

Hydration
Hydration is extremely important for humans. Water is used as a transportation device for nutrients, waste and hormones, is the main constituent of the human body, and also controls the acidity and electrolytes within cells. The main function of water, however, is to regulate body heat and temperature (thermo-regulation). Inadequate hydration will cause this temperature regulation to break down, which can lead to injury.

Humans generate their own body heat and they typically maintain a constant core temperature above environmental temperature. The heat to keep the body's temperature higher than the environmental temperature is produced metabolically. When the metabolic rate rises, heat production will increase, which in turn will lead to a rise in body temperature.

Heat can be produced in three ways:

• by a change in behaviour, for example, starting to exercise or move;
• through a response from the autonomic nervous system, such as shivering;
• by adaptation such as climatization.

The behavioural aspect of heat production is relevant here, as is the way the body reacts in order to lose the heat that exercise produces. In order for the body temperature to remain the same, the heat produced metabolically through exercise must be lost, using the following methods: conduction and convection (heat is lost as it is passed to the surroundings, such as the air in the room); radiation (heat is lost by producing infrared radiation); evaporation (sweat is produced and evaporates, resulting in a cooling effect). It is important to realize that, depending on the environment, conduction, convection and radiation may also increase the body temperature. This will occur when the temperature of the environment is higher than that of the body.

During training, an increase in body heat is produced, which upsets the heat balance, as heat production is higher than heat loss. The body will initiate autonomic heat-loss mechanisms (involuntary functions caused by the autonomic nervous system) to counter this heat production. These mechanisms will increase conduction of heat away from the core, so it can be lost through convection, radiation and/or evaporation. If these heat-loss mechanisms cannot cope with the increase in heat production, the body temperature will rise, which could ultimately lead to heat exhaustion.

About seventy-five to eighty per cent of the energy used by muscles is lost as heat. The total amount of heat produced is therefore closely related to the exercise intensity. The more physically demanding a martial arts class, the more energy will be used by the students and the more heat they will produce. This is a problem, especially in high-intensity exercise. This type of exercise generates a high demand for blood flow to the muscles to provide them with the necessary fuel. However, due to the intensity of the exercise and the heat produced by it, there is also a need for blood flow to the skin to promote heat loss. If the heart is unable to pump the blood around the body fast enough to provide for both (sufficient blood flow to muscles to keep exercising and sufficient blood flow to the skin to promote heat loss), the latter will be compromised. This will lead to reduced heat loss and a rapid rise in body temperature. Heat-loss mechanisms will be progressively impeded, leading to hyperthermia (over-heating), which will cause an individual to stop exercising.

Loss of performance can also be due to motivational factors, as some people are psychologically less tolerant of heat. More often, though, it is the result of competing demands in circulation to working muscles and to the skin.

Generally speaking, the body loses up to sixty per cent of its heat through radiation, and twelve to fifteen per cent through convection. The most efficient method of heat loss, however, is evaporation. At rest, without sweating, the body still loses about twenty-five percent of its heat through evaporation by means of respiration and body cavities. It is therefore important that students and/or fighters are adequately hydrated in order for their thermo-regulation to continue. Most heat delivered to the skin is lost by evaporation. The heat lost when sweat evaporation is maximal is less than the heat that is produced during high-intensity exercise – the body is able to produce heat faster than it can lose it.

Martial arts training usually takes place inside, in a comfortable ambient temperature and humidity. Even under these circumstances, sweat is often produced faster than evaporation takes place. However, in a full class, with a group of people exercising for a prolonged period, the temperature and humidity of a room can increase. The room becomes hot and the air very humid. Fluid loss becomes very apparent in these conditions because the effectiveness of evaporative cooling is hindered. The excessive output of sweat contributes little to cooling because evaporation is at a minimum. If this fluid could evaporate, it would at least have a cooling effect. However, in a hot and humid environment, radiation is not very effective and evaporation is not possible. Fluid is lost without the cooling effect; sweat will drip off the body without being any use to heat loss; sweat that is absorbed by clothing cannot evaporate and will not contribute to heat loss.

Losing fluid in this way will result in dehydration unless the right quantity of water is drunk. A prolonged martial arts class in the heat can lead to individuals losing more than two litres of body fluids per hour. Performance can suffer if as little as two per cent of body weight is lost through dehydration. If dehydration is over two per cent, the heart rate and body temperature become elevated during exercise. The increased heart rate is due to reduced central blood volume, which causes less blood to be pumped by the heart per beat; the heart compensates by beating more often. As dehydration progresses and more fluid is lost, the blood volume will drop and the blood will become more concentrated, sweating will be reduced and thermo-regulation will become progressively more difficult.

In this situation, performance will be badly affected. If fluid is not replaced, the reduction in circulatory fluid (blood) will mean less blood supply to exercising muscles, limiting the carbohydrate available as fuel, and less blood supply to the skin, thereby compromising heat loss. In order to sustain a high rate of work output in these conditions, the replacement of lost fluids is essential. As fluid is lost, sweating can no longer occur and the heat-loss mechanism will collapse. Dehydration and hyperthermia therefore go hand in hand. If an individual is insufficiently hydrated, his heat-loss capacity is impaired and hyperthermia will set in at an earlier stage.

Dehydration can have the following results:

- hyperthermia and reduced tolerance to heat stress;
- central fatigue due to the discomfort of being hot;
- circulatory alterations resulting in elevated heart rate;
- alterations in the mechanism of muscle contraction;
- increased risk of muscle damage, which will hamper recovery;
- increased rate of carbohydrate utilization, which could lead to a glycogen-depleted state;
- sweat gland fatigue, which could lead to reduction in the heat lost.

Fluid replacement during exercise is highly dependent on the rate of gastric emptying. During exercise gastric emptying is not halted. The stomach cannot let through matter of a higher consistency, but fluid replacement will still take place as this does not require much gastric activity. Water or any other liquid will pass quite readily through the stomach and small intestine in order to be absorbed. Fluid replacement will only reduce dehydration, it will not prevent it. Nevertheless, drinking during exercise will allow performance to be maintained for longer.

When teaching classes, the instructor must be very aware of the intensity of exercise and the fitness levels of the students. Sparring practice, repetitive techniques or combinations can all lead to high heat production. Water breaks must be incorporated, especially if training in a hot and/or humid environment. Venues for tournaments tend to be hot and/or humid, particularly if floodlighting is used and there is a big crowd present. Inadequate hydration leads to a drop in performance and a drop in concentration. This can lead to heat exhaustion, which is dangerous on its own. Diminished performance and concentration can lead to poor technique in the execution of skills, and the execution of technically and mechanically incorrect moves or combinations can cause injury.

If the exercise duration exceeds forty minutes (and martial arts classes generally do), the martial artist must begin fully hydrated and fluid levels must be kept up, especially in hot and humid conditions. Care must be taken to drink before the onset of thirst, as this sensation occurs in some people only after two per cent of the body weight has already been lost.

4 Body Basics

The Blood

The main role of the blood is to transport oxygen and nutrients around the body – an essential process for the function of all living cells. The cells of the body metabolize these nutrients to produce energy. An inevitable consequence of metabolism is the production of waste products, which are transported in the blood to the lungs and kidneys to be excreted. When the body is exercised, it requires more energy and therefore a greater supply of nutrients. The heart rate increases during exercise, increasing the blood supply to the muscles, allowing the rate of metabolism to rise. Consequently, the body produces more waste products during exercise than at rest.

Blood travels around the body through vessels known as arteries and veins. The arteries carry blood directly from the heart, which acts as a pump. As a result, the blood travelling through arteries is under high pressure. Veins return blood from the muscles and other organs back to the heart, and this blood is under lower pressure. The structure of arteries and veins differs to reflect the varying blood pressures within them. Arteries have thick walls containing a muscular layer, whereas the walls of veins are thinner and less muscular.

Once the tissues of the body have utilized the oxygen and nutrients within the blood, the blood must be returned to the lungs to be re-oxygenated. It is pumped by the heart through the lungs, which are the organs of gas exchange. Oxygen taken in with each breath diffuses from the lungs, through the blood-vessel walls, and into the blood. At the same time, carbon dioxide diffuses in the opposite direction, and is exhaled with each breath.

Bleeding

Bleeding results from damage to the blood vessels. Two types of bleeding can occur: *internal* and *external*. In internal bleeding, blood is lost into the cavities of the body. There are three main places where internal bleeding can occur:

- an injury to the chest can result in a broken rib and the sharp ends of a broken rib can cause damage to the underlying lung tissue. If a martial artist suffers such an injury and then coughs up blood, damage to the lung must be suspected. Blood can also collect within the cavity of the chest – the only signs of such an injury may be rapid breathing as the casualty goes into shock;
- an injury to the abdomen may also damage internal organs. The spleen is particularly susceptible when injuries occur to the left side of the abdomen. This is a medical emergency, as the spleen has a tendency to bleed profusely, which can rapidly lead to shock, and death. The liver can also be damaged by blows to the upper right aspect of the abdomen, but it is better protected by the ribcage than the spleen. Bleeding within

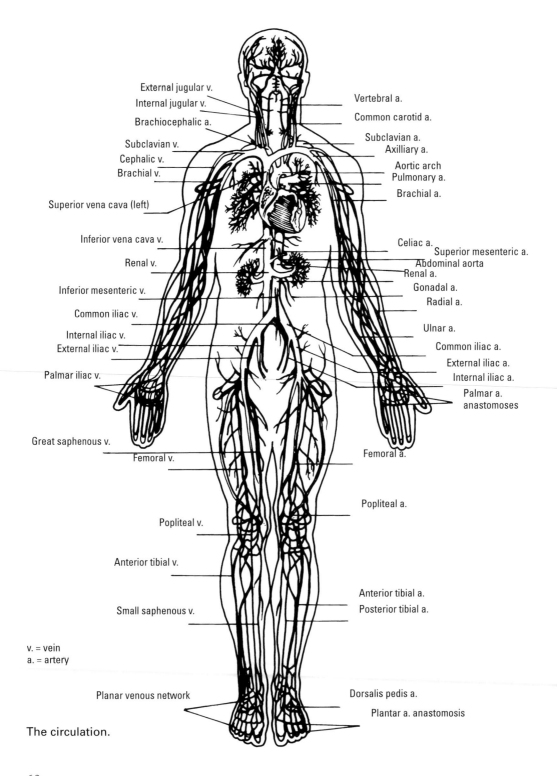

External jugular v.
Internal jugular v.
Brachiocephalic a.
Subclavian v.
Cephalic v.
Brachial v.
Superior vena cava (left)
Inferior vena cava v.
Renal v.
Inferior mesenteric v.
Common iliac v.
Internal iliac v.
External iliac v.
Palmar iliac v.
Great saphenous v.
Femoral v.
Popliteal v.
Anterior tibial v.
Small saphenous v.

Vertebral a.
Common carotid a.
Subclavian a.
Axilliary a.
Aortic arch
Pulmonary a.
Brachial a.
Celiac a.
Superior mesenteric a.
Abdominal aorta
Renal a.
Gonadal a.
Radial a.
Ulnar a.
Common iliac a.
External iliac a.
Internal iliac a.
Palmar a.
anastomoses
Femoral a.
Popliteal a.
Anterior tibial a.
Posterior tibial a.

v. = vein
a. = artery

Planar venous network

Dorsalis pedis a.
Plantar a. anastomosis

The circulation.

the abdomen and pelvis is extremely serious as there is a great deal of space for blood to collect, and surgery may be the only means of stopping the bleed;

- occasionally, certain injuries to other parts of the body, such as a fracture of the femur (thigh bone), can be associated with a significant amount of internal bleeding.

Internal bleeding can be a medical emergency – a person suffering from severe internal bleeding may very quickly go into shock and requires urgent medical attention.

External bleeding occurs as a result of a break in the skin and is visible. When severe, it is just as dangerous as internal bleeding. As the blood transported through arteries is under high pressure, damage to arteries can result in rapid blood loss. Blood loss from wounds must be controlled quickly by applying direct pressure to the wound. In healthy people, bleeding from superficial wounds should stop quickly, as blood exposed to the air clots to form a scab. Problems with the clotting process occur in certain medical conditions, resulting in a tendency to bruise, and prolonged bleeding.

Blood-Borne Diseases

First aiders must always be aware of the potential risks to themselves whenever considering action, including the transmission of blood-borne diseases from the injured person. Among the most serious of these diseases are HIV (Human Immuno-deficiency Virus) and Hepatitis. The risk of being infected with such a disease is extremely low – for such an infection to be transmitted, the infected blood must enter the first aider's bloodstream via an open wound or cut – and, indeed, there have been no reported cases of HIV or Hepatitis B transmitted during CPR (cardiopulmonary

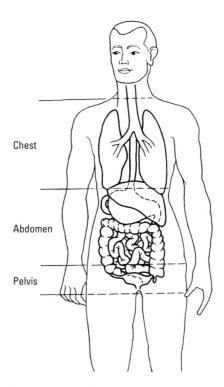

Chest

Abdomen

Pelvis

Sites of internal bleeding – chest, abdomen, pelvis.

resuscitation), but it is essential to minimize the risk as much as possible.

Disposable gloves are an essential part of a first aid kit, and it is advisable to wear them when dealing with any bleeding wound, and any other body fluid such as saliva or vomit. Similarly, any spillage of blood on to a training surface should be cleaned immediately with disinfectant, especially if martial artists using the area are training barefoot. In the competitive arena a fight should be stopped whenever a martial artist sustains a bleeding injury, so that it can be dealt with straight away.

Brain and Nerves

The nervous system can be divided into two parts: the *central nervous system* (CNS) and

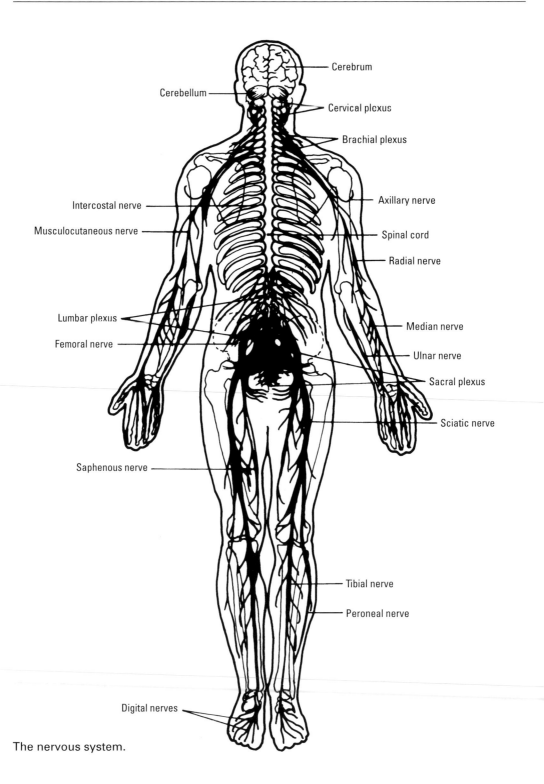

Cerebrum

Cerebellum

Cervical plexus

Brachial plexus

Intercostal nerve

Musculocutaneous nerve

Axillary nerve

Spinal cord

Radial nerve

Lumbar plexus

Femoral nerve

Median nerve

Ulnar nerve

Sacral plexus

Sciatic nerve

Saphenous nerve

Tibial nerve

Peroneal nerve

Digital nerves

The nervous system.

the *peripheral nervous system* (PNS). The CNS is made up of the brain and spinal cord, whereas the PNS comprises the nerves to the muscles and bones of the limbs.

The brain can be considered to be the control centre of the body, managing all of the body's functions, from breathing to walking. Messages from the brain are transmitted through nerves via the spinal cord to the muscles, bones and organs of the body. At the same time, nerves travel in the opposite direction – from the muscles and organs back to the brain. This system allows the brain to be constantly updated about the status of the body.

Injuries to the brain and spine can be fatal. Severe injury may result in a loss of breathing as the muscles responsible for respiration become paralysed, and death can follow swiftly. It is therefore of paramount importance that any person suspected of having sustained a head, neck, or spinal injury is managed quickly and effectively. Always suspect a neck or spinal injury when a casualty is found unconscious, or when a martial artist sustains a serious head injury.

The nerves of the body can be considered in terms of their function. Motor nerves carry messages from the brain and spinal cord to the muscles, in order to bring about movement. Sensory nerves carry messages in the opposite direction, constantly updating the brain as to the status of the body. Sensory nerves can be specialized to provide particular information – they may have receptors for the detection of pain, temperature, vibration and also the position of joints in space.

Nerves can be damaged as a result of injuries to the limbs and body, and certain nerves are particularly susceptible to damage because of their location. For example, injuries to the elbow place the ulnar nerve at risk of damage. Features of nerve injury include loss of movement in a particular part

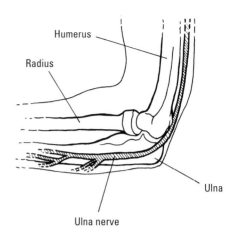

The relationship of the ulna nerve to the elbow.

of the body, as well as altered feelings in the skin, such as burning or tingling sensations. Damage to the nerves of the limbs can result in long-term loss of function. If a nerve is crushed, it is likely that there will be some re-growth and regeneration. If, on the other hand, a nerve is cut or 'transected', it is very rare for it to recover fully, even after surgical repair.

Muscles

The muscles of the body can be divided into two broad categories: *smooth muscle* and *skeletal muscle*. Smooth muscle cannot be controlled consciously. It is found in the walls of blood vessels and the intestines. The skeletal muscles of the body are essentially responsible for movement, and as such they act across the joints of the body. Muscles derive energy for movement by metabolizing oxygen and nutrients. As a result, skeletal muscles have a rich blood supply. The exact cause of muscle cramps is unknown, but one theory suggests that a cramp occurs when the blood supply to a muscle is inadequate to maintain its demand for oxygen and nutrients. Skeletal muscle has its own store

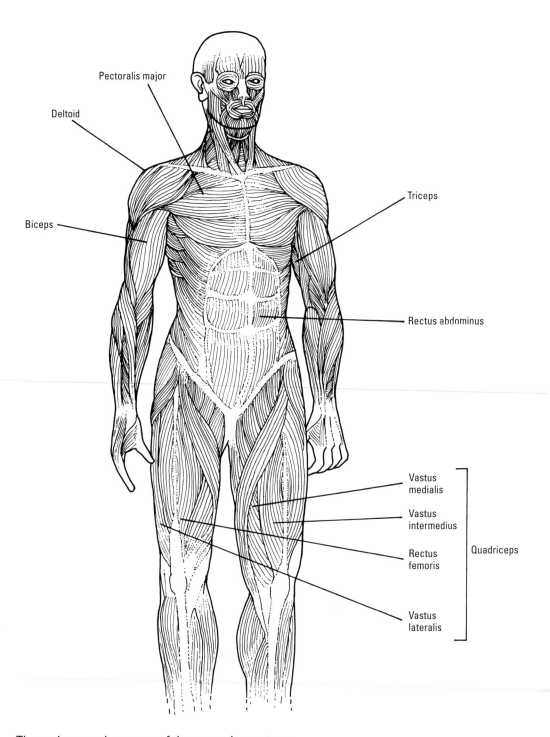

Pectoralis major

Deltoid

Biceps

Triceps

Rectus abdominus

Vastus
medialis

Vastus
intermedius

Rectus
femoris

Quadriceps

Vastus
lateralis

The major muscle groups of the muscular system.

of glucose in the form of glycogen. Glycogen is a complex carbohydrate which is broken down into glucose when muscles are exercised.

The muscles are also supplied by nerves from the brain and spinal cord, which allow the individual consciously to control the body's movement. If the nerve supply to a muscle is damaged, the muscle will waste away. The fibrous attachments of muscles to bone are known as tendons. Within the tendons there are specialized nerves, which constantly provide the central nervous system with information about the position of joints and limbs in space, in a process known as proprioception.

The skeletal muscles are made up of many individual muscle fibres. There are several types of muscle fibre, which differ in their speed of contractions, and also in endurance. These muscle fibres act as groups or units, and either contract or relax to cause movement.

Muscle strains occur when fibres are overstretched or torn. As with other injuries, these tears result in localized bleeding and the formation of blood clots. By applying ice to the torn muscle fibres and compressing the area, bleeding into the muscle can be reduced. At a later stage, it is possible to aid the breakdown of these blood clots, and also to promote healing, by applying heat and massaging the muscle.

Muscles can begin to ache and feel sore hours or days after exercising, especially when a person is unaccustomed to such exercise or when a training session has been particularly intense. This phenomenon is known as 'delayed onset muscle soreness', or DOMS. The soreness and aching may continue to increase even without further training, reaching a maximum at one or two days after the initial bout of exercise. This occurs as a result of reversible damage to and swelling within the muscle fibres.

Someone suffering from DOMS may also feel as though the muscles are weaker. In general, this muscle damage is fully reversed within about ten days, and for this reason it is essential that a martial artist has adequate rest periods in between intense training sessions. If exercise of a similar intensity is repeated, the muscles sustain less damage, which means that the individual can adapt and become more resistant to heavy training schedules.

Skeletal System

The structure of the bones that form the skeleton is extremely complex. The core of long bones, such as the femur (thigh bone), is made up of a complicated network of materials, which include calcium. Around this core there is more dense bone, which gives the skeleton strength and stability. The structure of the skeleton is not static – bones are constantly changing and being remodelled. Bones are also surrounded by a covering containing arteries and nerves – damage to this covering layer will result in the death of the underlying bone.

In order for a broken bone to heal correctly, the ends of the bone must be placed in close apposition and the blood supply to the bone must be intact. It is therefore essential for all suspected fractures to be X-rayed so that it can be decided whether a plaster cast or surgery is required. If fractures are not managed correctly, the blood supply to the bone may remain obstructed, resulting in the death of the bone. One of the most serious complications of a fracture is bone infection. The risk of infection is high when a broken bone penetrates the skin, therefore exposing it to the environment. Such an injury must be covered with a sterile dressing as quickly as possible in order to minimize the risk of infection.

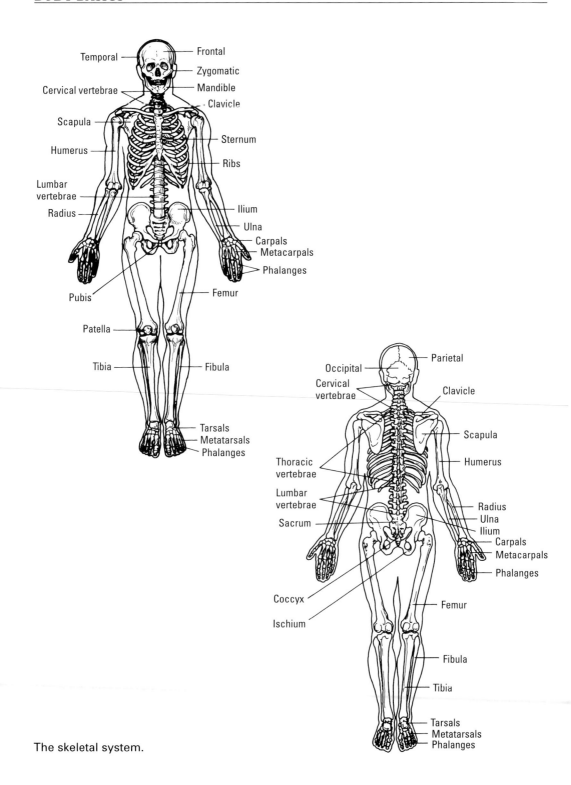

The skeletal system.

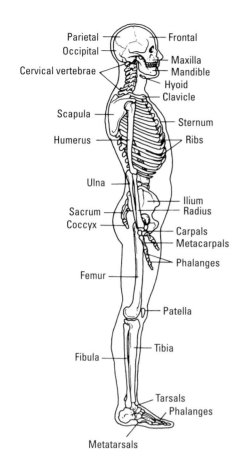

Parietal
Occipital
Cervical vertebrae
Scapula
Humerus
Ulna
Sacrum
Coccyx
Femur
Fibula
Metatarsals
Frontal
Maxilla
Mandible
Hyoid
Clavicle
Sternum
Ribs
Ilium
Radius
Carpals
Metacarpals
Phalanges
Patella
Tibia
Tarsals
Phalanges

Injury and Inflammation

When injuries to the muscles, bones and soft tissues occur, the body responds by acting to protect the injured area and also to promote healing. This natural mechanism is known as the *inflammatory response*. The characteristic features of inflammation are:

* swelling;
* pain;
* heat;
* redness.

Swelling

Injuries result in swelling through a variety of mechanisms. Swelling occurs because blood vessels become leaky, which can be a direct result of trauma or due to the release of chemicals from inflammatory cells in the area of the injury. As a consequence, fluid from within the blood vessels leaks into damaged tissue. This fluid is rich in proteins, nutrients and activated cells from within the blood, which are essential for tissue healing. As a rough guide, the greater the amount of swelling, the more serious an injury is likely to be.

Several simple measures can be employed to reduce swelling. First, elevate the injured body part to allow gravity to drain the fluid away. Second, apply ice wrapped in a cloth, or a cold compress, to reduce blood flow to the area and therefore reduce the leakage of fluid into the tissues. Third, compress the area, for example with an elasticated bandage, to help fluid to drain away from the injured area. Once inflammation begins to subside, it is advisable to begin gentle activity as soon as possible to prevent the stiffening up of joints and loss of movement.

These principles for the management of injury can be remembered by using the acronym PRICE: P – protect; R – rest; I – ice; C – compress; E – elevate.

Pain

Throughout the body there are specialized nerve endings that act as pain receptors. When soft tissues are damaged, pain is felt for a variety of reasons. First, the swelling associated with inflammation results in the stretching of pain receptors within the muscle, joint, joint capsule, bone or blood vessels. Second, there are several chemicals within the inflammatory fluid that act directly on nerve endings to cause the sensation of pain.

Pain is the body's natural alarm system for alerting you to injury. It should act as a reminder that an injured body part should first of all be protected, to prevent any further damage. Pain should never be ignored, especially when it is sufficient to prevent a person from functioning normally, for example, if it causes a limp, or disturbs sleep.

Heat and Redness

An injured joint or muscle may feel hot and appear red because of increased blood flow to the damaged tissues – in medical terms the area is hyperaemic. The increase in blood flow promotes healing by increasing the delivery of oxygen and nutrients, which are essential for rapid repair, and also allows efficient removal of the waste products of metabolism. Again, rest, ice, compression and elevation will help to reduce the heat and redness that results from injury.

Scarring

Scars occur as a result of the body's natural healing process. Scarring can be seen on the surface when skin heals, but also occurs when a muscle or ligament is torn. Scar tissue is more fibrous than the body tissue it replaces, and therefore less flexible. As a result, severe scarring can reduce the performance of muscles and ligaments.

Types of Injury

Cuts

A cut or laceration is an injury that involves a break in the skin. As with any bleeding injury, the first priority must be to stop bleeding by applying a clean dressing and direct pressure on to the area. Once bleeding is arrested, the wound should be cleaned thoroughly to reduce the risk of infection. A gaping wound should be assessed in

hospital, as the edges of a large wound must be held in close apposition in order to heal properly, and with minimal scarring. This may require stitches, glue or taping. If a martial artist sustains a cut to the scalp that bleeds profusely, a simple way of closing the wound is to take hair from either side of the cut and to tie it, bringing the edges of the wound together.

A break in the skin that occurs as a result of a human bite or catching the skin on an opponent's tooth requires medical attention. The mouth is naturally colonized by a whole host of bacteria, so any such wound must be cleaned effectively, and the casualty given antibiotics.

An insight into the anatomy of an area affected by a deep cut will allow the first aider to consider whether any underlying structures, such as nerves or blood vessels, could have been damaged.

Bruises

A bruise occurs as a result of the leakage of blood under the skin from damaged blood vessels. A bruise follows a characteristic sequence of colour changes. The initial red colour reflects the redness of oxygenated blood leaking from broken blood vessels. A bruise then becomes a darker blue-black colour as the blood becomes deoxygenated. Finally, the area turns a yellowish-green colour as the blood is broken down and reabsorbed. Applying an ice pack can reduce bruising by decreasing the blood flow to the area.

Muscle Strains

A strain occurs as a result of overstretching a muscle. Common contributing factors are inadequate warm-up routines and poor technique. To some extent, a muscle strain should be considered as a preventable injury. When a muscle fibre is torn, there is always some degree of bleeding and swelling. Blood clots form and the area is tender to the touch. After initially applying a cold pack to the area to reduce swelling and bleeding into the muscle, heat and massage can aid in the breakdown of blood clots, and therefore promote healing.

Sprains

A sprain describes an injury to a ligament, often as a result of overstretching. Ligaments attach from bone to bone, across a joint, and act to provide stability. A severe sprain can result in a joint becoming unstable, especially if a ligament is torn. It is important to recognize a sprained joint, as recovery can be a long process requiring physiotherapy and expert guidance.

Dislocation

A dislocation occurs when a bone is forced out of its normal alignment within a joint. Dislocations usually occur as a result of the application of considerable force to a joint. Some people are more prone to joint dislocations than others. When someone suffers a dislocated joint, it is likely that the ligaments have also been damaged as the ligaments play an important role in maintaining the stability of a joint. It is also common for fractures and dislocations to occur together – an injury known as a fracture-dislocation. A dislocation can also result in damage to nearby blood vessels and nerves.

Fracture

A fracture is the breakage of a bone, which may be complete or incomplete. Fractures are usually caused by direct forces acting on a bone, but can also occur as a result of twisting and indirect forces, as well as long-term stresses. A bone can also be fractured as a result of excess forces pulling on the bony attachment of a tendon; this injury is known as an avulsion fracture.

There are several important complications that can occur as a result of a fracture. A fractured bone that penetrates the skin is at risk of becoming infected. If a fractured bone is not managed correctly, it may heal out of line, resulting in deformity and loss of function. This is a particular risk when a fracture affects or is close to a joint. A fractured bone may also fail to heal at all, particularly if the blood supply is compromised. For these reasons, it is essential to have a low threshold of suspicion for a fracture. As a general rule, a fracture needs to be ruled out whenever an injury is sufficiently serious to cause pronounced swelling and bruising of a body part, and whenever an injury is sufficiently painful as to disrupt normal activities such as walking.

When a bone is fractured, it may be forced out of its normal alignment. As a consequence of this, any blood vessels or nerves that run in parallel to the bone are at risk of being damaged or obstructed. This complication can occur when the ankle is broken, in which case the blood and nerve supply to the foot is compromised.

Vascular Injuries

Vascular injuries, or injuries to blood vessels, are obvious when there is a visible site of bleeding. Compromise of the blood supply to a limb can also occur as a result of a fracture or dislocation, and in such a case vascular injury may be less obvious. When a limb is deprived of its arterial blood supply for more than a few minutes, the skin becomes pale, later appearing blue and mottled as tissues begin to die. The area may also feel numb and the casualty may complain of strange sensations such as tingling or burning. Any muscles that are supplied by the compromised blood vessels will become weak, and the pulses in the limb will be lost.

5 Shock

Shock can be considered as the body's response to severe trauma. There are four main categories, which are classified according to their cause:

1. *cardiogenic shock* – when the heart or circulatory system is severely compromised;
2. *septic shock* – due to an overwhelming infection;
3. *anaphylactic shock* – due to an excessive allergic response;
4. *neurogenic shock* – due to compromise of the central nervous system.

Shock, in the context of first aid, is most likely to be cardiogenic and the result of severe blood loss. The features of shock arise as a result of the body's attempt to ensure that the brain is able to function in spite of severe injury or blood loss.

The Circulatory System

Every living tissue within the body requires oxygen and nutrients to survive. Blood is pumped around the body by the heart in order to deliver these substances. As the brain is essentially the body's control centre, it is vital that the brain receives an adequate blood supply at all times. The circulatory system can be compromised by damage to any part of the circuit:

- the heart, as in, for example, a heart attack;

- the blood vessels, when there is, for example, a blockage as a result of a blood clot;
- severe blood loss.

When the circulatory system is compromised to such an extent that it can no longer compensate for the damage, the body acts to protect the blood supply to the brain. It does this by diverting blood away from the limbs and organs of the body, and transporting this blood to the brain. The features that result from the diversion of blood are known collectively as *shock*.

Recognizing Shock

There are a number of distinguishing features associated with shock:

- the casualty becomes pale, cold and clammy as blood is diverted away from the skin;
- breathing becomes more rapid and shallow;
- the injured person may vomit or feel nauseous;
- initially the casualty's pulse rate will be rapid – if the casualty continues to deteriorate the pulse will slow;
- as the blood supply to the brain begins to fail, the person may become restless and angry;
- eventually the casualty will lose consciousness and the heart will stop beating.

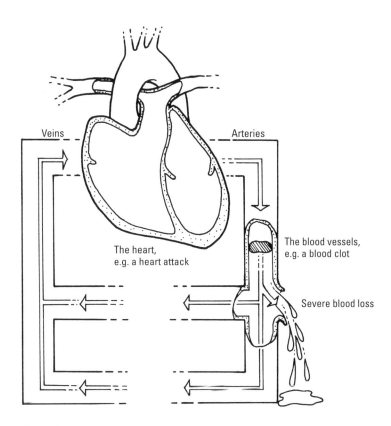

Veins

Arteries

The heart,
e.g. a heart attack

The blood vessels,
e.g. a blood clot

Severe blood loss

Causes of
circulatory shock

The earlier the signs of shock are recognized, the earlier the casualty can be treated. In the context of martial arts, shock is most likely to occur from an injury resulting in severe internal or external bleeding. A fracture of the long bones of the leg, or a severe abdominal injury may cause such bleeding. Other causes of circulatory failure include a heart attack and a blood clot in the lung, which is also known as a pulmonary embolism. Both of these conditions are more common with age.

Monitoring a Casualty

It is possible to monitor the status of a casualty who has sustained a severe injury by recording their breathing and pulse rates. The breathing and pulse rates differ from person to person, but as a guide, a normal breathing rate is between twelve and sixteen breaths per minute, and a normal pulse rate between sixty and 100 beats per minute.

To record the breathing rate:

1. observe the rise and fall of the chest with each breath;
2. count how many breaths the casualty takes in fifteen seconds;
3. multiply this number by four in order to calculate the breathing rate per minute;
4. as shock progresses, the breathing rate will increase at first, then slow and eventually stop – the injured person may need resuscitation.

To record the pulse rate:

1. find the pulsation of the radial artery on the inside of the wrist with your first and

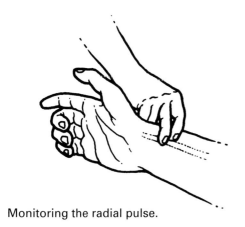

Monitoring the radial pulse.

second fingers – it can be found just above a tendon in the wrist, about 3cm (just over an inch) from the base of the thumb;

2. count the number of pulsations in fifteen seconds;
3. multiply this number by four to calculate the pulse rate per minute;
4. initially a shocked casualty will have a high pulse rate – later the pulse rate will

decrease as the heart begins to fail. If the heart stops you will have to carry out CPR (*see* page 00).

Anyone who is trained to do so can also monitor the carotid pulse in the neck.

FIRST AID FOR THE SHOCKED CASUALTY

1. Act as soon as you recognize the features of shock. Ask the casualty to lie down and raise their feet off the floor.
2. Identify any bleeding wounds and apply a dressing and direct pressure to stop the bleeding.
3. Cover the injured person with a blanket.
4. Send someone to call for the emergency services and ask for an ambulance.
5. While you wait for the ambulance, reassure the casualty, and remove any tight clothing from around the chest or neck.
6. Monitor the casualty's breathing and pulse rate at one-minute intervals – be ready to perform resuscitation if the breathing or pulse stops.

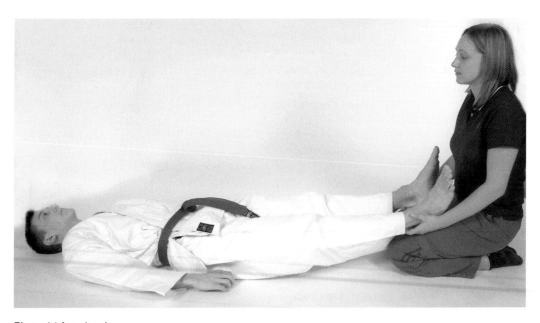

First aid for shock.

6 Essential First Aid

The Unconscious Casualty

A martial artist may become unconscious for a number of reasons. An injury to the head may cause a loss of consciousness – usually just for a short time – while a more serious injury may cause a more prolonged period of unconsciousness, and requires immediate attention. A person may also lose consciousness for reasons unrelated to martial arts training – for example, in the case of a heart attack. When the body is awake and alert, natural reflexes act to protect the airways. These reflexes are lost when a person becomes unconscious, resulting in the airway becoming obstructed.

Before approaching the casualty, *make sure that it is safe* to do so – risks include sharp objects and electrical equipment. There is no sense in creating two casualties by injuring yourself.

If a martial artist does become unconscious, for any reason, it is essential to act quickly and appropriately. Always consider the possibility of a neck or spinal injury when a casualty is found unconscious. If you have witnessed the events leading to a martial artist becoming unconscious and consider a neck injury to be unlikely, follow the procedure below. If you are at all unsure, err on the side of caution and assess the casualty for a neck injury before moving the head.

In order to assess the unconscious casualty for head or neck injury, take the following steps:

1. take a step back from the casualty and consider whether the neck and spine appear in normal alignment;
2. examine the head and neck by gently feeling for swelling, sites of bleeding or depressions in the skull, taking care not to move the head;
3. inspect the ears and nose for any discharge of fluid or blood, which would indicate a possible skull fracture;
4. if the injured martial artist regains consciousness, ask whether he has any neck or back pain.

FIRST AID FOR THE UNCONSCIOUS CASUALTY, AND CPR

1. First check that the martial artist has actually lost consciousness and not just fainted. Call his name and shake him firmly by the shoulders, *unless you suspect a neck injury*. If you do suspect a neck injury, the casualty should not be moved.
2. If the casualty does not respond, the first priority is to call for help – send someone to call the emergency services and ask for an ambulance. If the casualty has had a heart attack and the heart stops beating, it is very unlikely that it will be possible to restart the heart without shocking or 'defibrillating' the patient.
3. Think of A, B, C: A – airway, B – breathing, C – circulation.
4. The next step is to open the injured casualty's *airway* (A). When a person loses consciousness it is possible for the tongue to fall backwards in the mouth

and therefore obstruct the airway. *Unless you suspect a neck or spinal injury,* tilt the casualty's head back by placing one hand on the forehead and the other under the chin. Then lift the chin by placing your fingers under the front of the jaw and lifting upwards.

5. After opening the airway, assess whether or not the casualty is *breathing* (B), using three methods – *look, listen and feel.* Turn your head and place your cheek over the casualty's mouth to feel for breathing on your cheek. At the same time, watch the chest to assess whether it is rising and falling. As you look and feel, listen for the casualty's breathing sounds. Assess the breathing for ten seconds. If the casualty is breathing normally, turn him over into the recovery position and wait for help to arrive. *If the casualty is not breathing you will have to breathe for him using mouth-to-mouth ventilation.*

6. To give mouth-to-mouth ventilation, place your mouth over the casualty's mouth forming a tight seal, and at the same time pinch the casualty's nose to prevent air from escaping. (A simple resuscitation device may be used over the casualty's mouth for reasons of hygiene, preventing direct contact.) Take a deep breath in, then give two rescue breaths by exhaling sharply into the casualty's mouth until the chest rises. Repeat the procedure for the second rescue breath when the chest has fallen, then assess the casualty's circulation.

7. If the rescue breaths are ineffective, look inside the mouth and remove any objects that could be obstructing the airway. Make sure that the head is tilted back and that the chin has been lifted. If after five attempts you still have not achieved two rescue breaths, move on to assessment of the circulation.

8. Assess the casualty's *circulation* (C) by feeling for the carotid pulse in the neck, *only if you are trained to do so.* If you are not trained to feel the carotid pulse, ask yourself the following questions: Is the casualty moving at all? Is the casualty coughing or making any other noises? Does the casualty appear pale and feel cold to the touch? Spend ten seconds assessing for signs of circulation. If you are confident that you can detect signs of circulation, continue rescue breaths until the casualty begins to breathe.

9. If the casualty is not moving, is not making any sounds, and appears pale and cold, proceed to chest compressions.

10. To perform chest compressions, find the casualty's breastbone (sternum) and follow it towards the legs until you come to its end, just above the abdomen. Place two fingers side by side at the end of the breastbone, then place the heel of one hand above your two fingers. Place one hand on top of the other and interlock your fingers. Compress the chest approximately 4–5cm (1½–2in) fifteen times, aiming for a rate of 100 compressions per minute.

11. After fifteen compressions, re-check the breathing and circulation. If there is no change, give two more breaths and fifteen chest compressions.

12. Re-assess the breathing and circulation after every cycle of two breaths and fifteen compressions. Continue CPR until help arrives, or until the casualty shows signs of life.

If you are unable to give the casualty rescue breaths for any reason, or if there is blood or vomit around the mouth, carry out chest compressions without rescue breaths in between. There is some evidence that chest compressions alone are beneficial to a casualty who is not breathing.

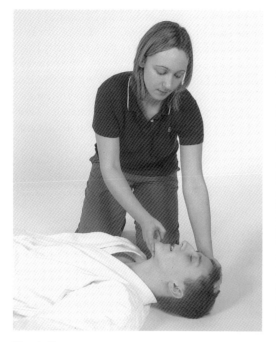

Head tilt.

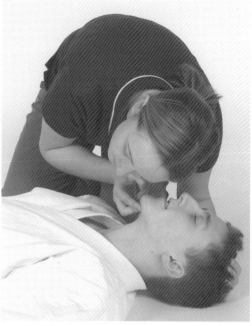

Assessment of breathing.

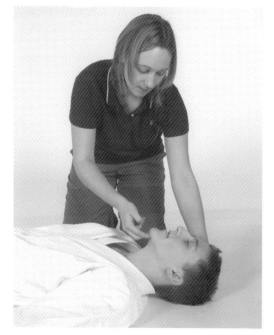

Chin lift.

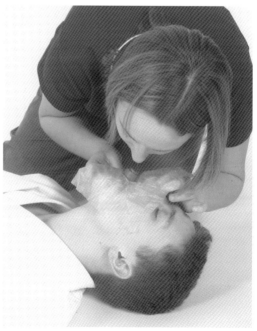

Resuscitation with a device.

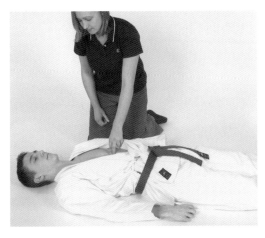

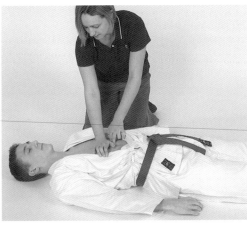

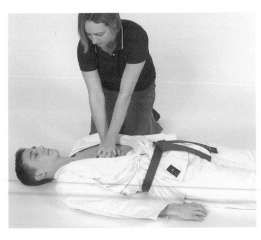

Chest compressions.

If there is more than one person present with the casualty, two-person CPR is possible. The first person gives the two rescue breaths, followed by the second person giving fifteen chest compressions. If CPR must be continued for a prolonged period, the two people can alternate their roles at regular intervals, in order to prevent fatigue.

Carrying out CPR is exhausting – if there are more people available, allow them to take over when you become tired.

The ABCs

Following the principles of A, B, C – airway, breathing, circulation – can save a life, but why are these procedures so important, and why are they done in this particular order?

The purpose of mouth-to-mouth resuscitation and chest compressions is to take over the role of the casualty's breathing and circulation, until definitive treatment can be given, or until the casualty recovers. The aim is to provide the brain with oxygenated blood so that it can continue to function. If the brain is starved of oxygen for more than three to four minutes, the casualty will suffer irreparable brain damage.

The airway is checked first for two reasons. First, an obstructed airway will result in death before compromised breathing or circulation, and second because an obstructed airway must be cleared before rescue breaths can be administered effectively. The next priority is to assess the breathing because it is necessary to ensure that oxygen is reaching the blood, before the blood is transported to the brain by the circulation.

Even when CPR is carried out effectively, it achieves a level of circulation that is only thirty per cent of the heart's normal activity. It is therefore essential to call for the emergency services as soon as possible. If a

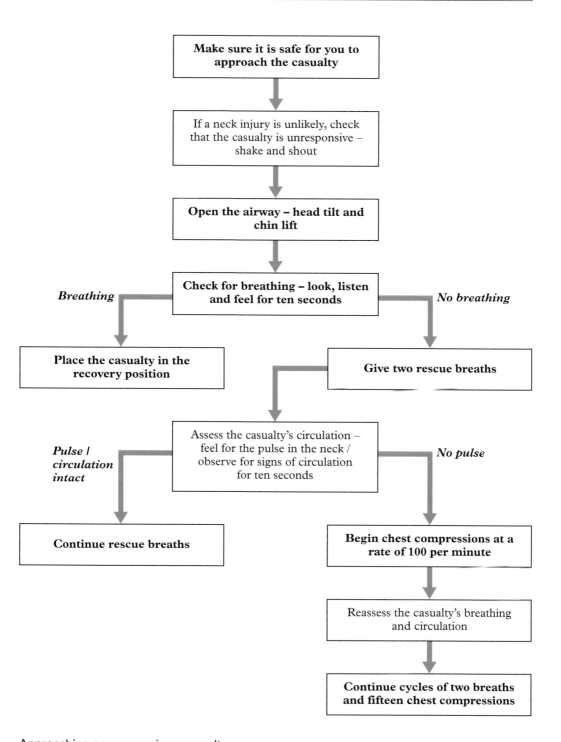

Approaching an unconscious casualty.

person's heart stops beating, it is unlikely that the heart will be restarted without electrical defibrillation.

The Recovery Position

This position helps an unconscious casualty to breathe by opening the airway and draining fluids from the nose and throat so they are not inhaled. This is the safest position for an unconscious casualty to be in if he is breathing, after you have called the emergency services and asked for an ambulance.

While a casualty is in the recovery position, waiting for help to arrive, it is essential that the vital signs are monitored. Regularly monitoring the casualty's breathing rate and pulse rate allows a quick reaction to any change.

Remember: do not move the casualty if you suspect that he has been seriously injured and may have sustained a neck injury.

To put the unconscious casualty who is

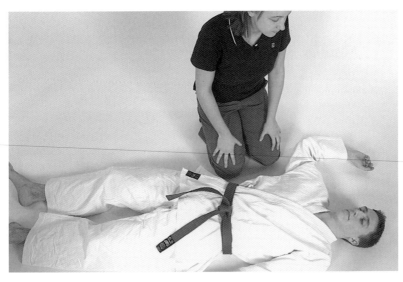

The recovery position.

1

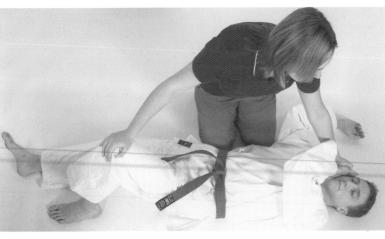

2

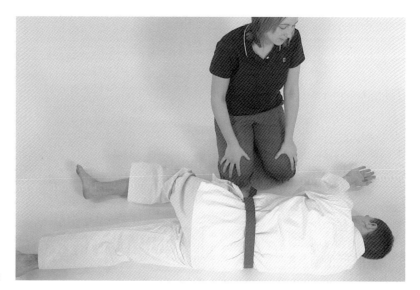

3

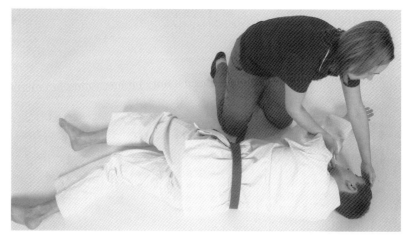

4

breathing into the recovery position, take the following steps:

1. kneel down next to the injured casualty. Take the arm nearest to you, and straighten it out at 90 degrees to the body with the palm of the hand facing up;
2. take the hand furthest from you and place the back of the hand against the casualty's cheek. Use your free hand to bend the leg furthest away from you;
3. use the casualty's bent leg as a lever to

pull the casualty over on to their side. Whilst holding the casualty's hand against his cheek, pull the leg towards you. Make sure that the casualty's head is resting on his own hand;
4. tilt the casualty's head back to open the airway;
5. regularly check the breathing and circulation until help arrives. Listen out for noisy breathing or any sign that the casualty's airway may be compromised.

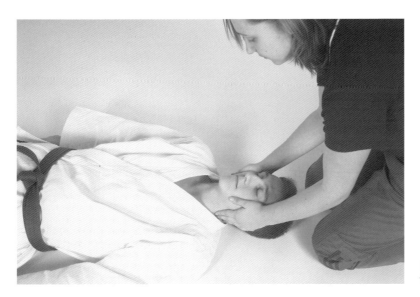

Immobilization of the neck.

Neck and Spinal Injury

Injury to the neck or spine is a medical emergency – if you suspect it, the first action must be to *call the emergency services and ask for an ambulance*. It is essential that the casualty is correctly managed until help arrives. There are certain key points to remember:

1. do not move a casualty if you suspect a neck or spine injury;
2. if you must carry out CPR, use the jaw thrust technique to open the airway and not the head tilt (see the picture opposite);
3. always suspect a neck injury when a casualty has sustained an injury to the head.

Any sudden movements of the spine or neck could result in paralysis or even death, as a fractured bone may be displaced and sever the spinal cord. Transporting a casualty with a spinal injury should be left to paramedics or other medically trained personnel who will stabilize the neck and spine before any movement.

If the casualty is conscious, he must be told to remain completely still. There are a number of clues to the fact that a martial artist may be suffering a spinal cord injury. He may complain of some or all of the following:

• weakness or inability to move the fingers or toes;
• feelings of numbness or tingling in the arms or legs;
• severe pain along the line of the spine, or shooting pains along the limbs.

In addition, the appearance of the spine may be altered or 'out of line'.

FIRST AID FOR NECK INJURIES

To deal with a casualty with a neck injury who is *conscious*, proceed as follows:

1. tell the injured person to try to remain as still as possible;
2. the main priority is to *immobilize the casualty's neck and spine*. Using one hand on either side of the injured person's head, hold it completely still in the position in which the casualty was found;

3. to immobilize the spine, place rolled-up towels on either side of the neck, to prevent any movement;
4. monitor the casualty's breathing and circulation until help arrives – you may have to carry out CPR.

To deal with a casualty with a neck injury who is *unconscious*, proceed as follows:

1. the first priority is to assess the casualty's airway, breathing and circulation;
2. if the casualty is *unconscious but breathing*, the next step is to immobilize the neck and spine;
3. using one hand on either side of the head, hold the head still in the position in which the injured person is lying. Alternatively, place rolled-up towels on either side of the head to prevent any movement of the head and neck;
4. monitor the casualty's breathing and circulation until help arrives;
5. if the casualty is *unconscious and not breathing* you must open the airway without moving the casualty's neck. Place the first two fingers of each hand behind the angles of the casualty's jaw. Use your fingers to apply steady pressure upwards

and forwards, and use your thumbs to open the mouth. This manoeuvre is known as the *jaw thrust*, and should always be used if you suspect that a casualty has sustained a neck injury;
6. perform two rescue breaths and then go on to assess the casualty's circulation. If you cannot feel a pulse, perform CPR. *At all times be aware that the neck and spine must remain immobile.*

The First Aid Kit

A well-stocked first aid kit must be available at all venues where martial arts are practised, and where competitions are held. Ready-prepared first aid kits are available from chemists and other shops. Most contain sufficient supplies to deal with the minor problems that commonly occur during the course of everyday life. A good way to make sure that your first aid kit has the correct equipment to deal with the majority of martial arts injuries is to go through a list and consider what is required to deal effectively with each type of injury. It is also important to re-check the first aid kit at regular intervals, in case any stock needs to be replaced.

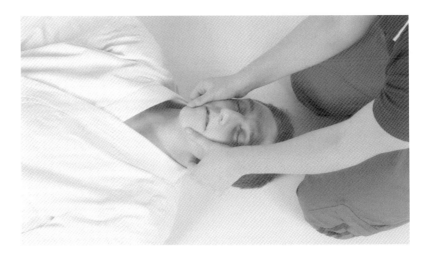

The jaw thrust.

First aid kit checklist

- sterile swabs or gauze pads;
- sterile wound dressings and plasters;
- compressive bandages;
- triangular bandages;
- antiseptic cream;
- disposable gloves;
- mask device for mouth-to-mouth ventilation.

Key principles for the first aider

- Before approaching a casualty, make sure that it is safe to do so.
- Make a quick assessment of the seriousness of the situation; be ready to call for help at an early stage.
- Try to remain calm – this is of particular importance in certain injuries, such as injuries of the throat, when it is essential to reassure the casualty so that he also remains calm.
- Stick to the basics – remember the A, B, C of life support. Assessment of airway, breathing and circulation should always come first – do not be sidetracked by other injuries.
- Take a moment to consider the mechanism of the injury – if the injured fighter has sustained a head injury, ask yourself whether the neck may also have been damaged.
- If you suspect that the injured martial artist has sustained a neck injury, the neck must be immobilized – do not move the casualty
- Never do anything that you feel uncomfortable doing or that you have not been trained to do – you may do more harm than good.
- There is no substitute for practice – regularly update and refresh your first aid skills by attending courses.

Perhaps the most important piece of equipment is a phone, so that the emergency services can be called at the earliest opportunity. Ice is also important – many sports centres are equipped with ice machines, but ice may be less easily available at other martial arts venues. A special mask device will prevent direct physical contact with a casualty during resuscitation. This will be particularly useful when there is blood or vomit in the casualty's mouth.

First Aid Equipment for Various Injuries

Cuts, Grazes and Other Superficial Wounds

An injury that results in a break in the skin will require thorough cleaning, and if bleeding is prominent, direct pressure will be required. Always wear disposable gloves when dealing with blood. Place sterile dressings over the wound then apply pressure with a hand. Once bleeding has stopped, the area should be cleaned under running water.

Before dressing a superficial wound, it is advisable to apply an antiseptic cream to reduce the risk of infection. If a wound continues to bleed, apply a dressing then maintain pressure by wrapping a compressive bandage around the bleeding limb and transport the casualty to hospital.

Remember to disinfect any areas of the practice arena where blood has been spilt, in order to protect other martial artists.

Bruises, Sprains and Strains

As with other soft-tissue injuries, a cold compress or ice wrapped in a cloth should be applied to the area. The ice should be changed every fifteen to twenty minutes for up to two hours. Ice should not be placed in direct contact with the skin. Once swelling has reduced, a warm compress may help to ease pain.

Fractures and Dislocations

It is useful to have a supply of soft material to wrap around injured limbs and joints to prevent further damage to the area. Keep at least two large triangular bandages in the first aid kit in order to make a sling and also to immobilize broken limbs.

7 Head and Facial Injuries

Injuries to the head can be sustained when a martial artist is thrown or swept on to a hard surface. Direct blows to the head can also cause injury. Head injuries require particular attention, as some serious ones can lead to the rapid deterioration of the subject's health. It is also important to realize that some injuries can cause bleeding within the skull, resulting in the slow accumulation of blood. In such a case, the signs of injury may only become apparent hours after the initial injury. Bleeding within the skull is particularly common when blows to the side of the head are sustained.

Whenever a martial artist sustains a head injury, you must consider the possibility of a concurrent neck or spinal injury. (Training to improve the strength and tone of the neck muscles can help to reduce the risk of neck injuries. If a blow to the head is sustained while the neck muscles are tensed, some of the force will be absorbed by the muscles and transferred to the trunk.)

A head injury may result in a cut to the scalp, which can bleed surprisingly heavily, because the scalp has a rich blood supply. As with other bleeding wounds, applying direct pressure will help to stop the flow. The brain is suspended within the skull, and a blow to the head can cause concussion – a brief period of unconsciousness when the brain is shaken (*see* below).

The skull bones may be fractured by a particularly heavy impact. Skull fractures are particularly important to identify because there may be damage to underlying brain tissue. Furthermore, if there is an open wound over a fracture site, it is possible for infection to reach the central nervous system from the outside environment.

Alternatively, the blood vessels within the skull and brain may be damaged, leading to unseen bleeding, which can increase the pressure within the skull, and cause the casualty's conscious level to deteriorate. Bleeding within the brain is a condition which can be rapidly fatal without surgery.

Assessment and Recognition

When dealing with someone who has suffered a head injury, you should take the following steps:

1. *call for help* if you suspect a serious head injury;
2. if the injured martial artist is unconscious, assess their breathing and circulation;
3. if you suspect a neck or spinal injury, do not move the casualty – follow the procedure given on page 80.

A casualty suffering a serious head injury requiring medical attention may display the following features:

- loss of consciousness, confusion or drowsiness;
- weakness or inability to move any part of the body;

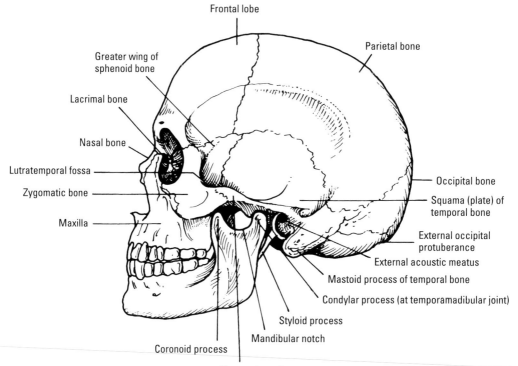

Frontal lobe

Parietal bone

Greater wing of
sphenoid bone

Lacrimal bone

Nasal bone

Lutratemporal fossa

Zygomatic bone

Maxilla

Occipital bone

Squama (plate) of
temporal bone

External occipital
protuberance

External acoustic meatus

Mastoid process of temporal bone

Condylar process (at temporamadibular joint)

Styloid process

Mandibular notch

Coronoid process

Zygomatic arch

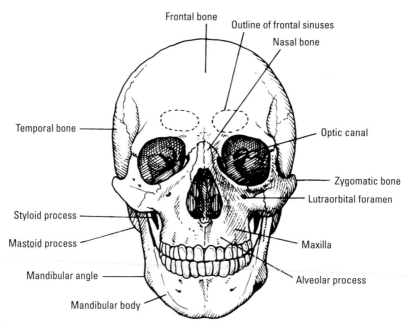

Frontal bone

Outline of frontal sinuses

Nasal bone

Temporal bone

Optic canal

Zygomatic bone

Lutraorbital foramen

Styloid process

Mastoid process

Maxilla

Mandibular angle

Alveolar process

Mandibular body

The skull.

- convulsions (fits or seizures);
- loss of vision, blurred or double vision, or pupils of unequal size;
- deformity or depression of the skull;
- blood or fluid draining from the mouth, nose or ears;
- severe headache or vomiting.

Types of Head Injury

Concussion

A blow to the head may cause the brain to be shaken within the confines of the skull. This disturbance is known as a concussion, and is characterized by a brief loss of consciousness followed by complete recovery. A severe concussion can result in a prolonged period of unconsciousness, but it is more common for a casualty to recover quickly. If you suspect that someone has suffered a concussion, ask the person a few basic questions – if the casualty cannot remember simple information, such as his own name, or where he is, further assessment is required.

Concussion may be indicated by the following features:

- a brief period of unconsciousness following a blow to the head;
- some dizziness or nausea, and the casualty may even vomit;
- the casualty may suffer a mild headache after the incident.

FIRST AID FOR HEAD INJURY

1. If the casualty is unconscious, place him in the recovery position. Work quickly if he is vomiting.
2. Monitor and record the casualty's breathing and pulse rate. If he does not regain consciousness within *three minutes*, suspect a more serious injury. Send someone to *call the emergency services and ask for an ambulance*.

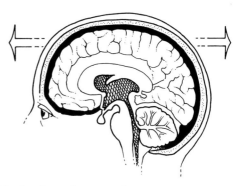

Mechanism of concussion.

3. If the casualty recovers within three minutes, observe him closely for any change in the level of consciousness. A concussed martial artist should not be allowed to continue the training session, even if he appears to recover.

The injured person should seek medical attention if they continue to suffer from headache, nausea, drowsiness or any of the problems mentioned above.

Concussions are classified medically according to their severity. A martial artist suffering a concussion should seek professional advice on how long to refrain from training after such an injury. The usual time allowed for recovery from a mild concussion is between one week and one month. More severe concussions require a longer recovery period, and it is essential that a martial artist has been symptom-free for some time before returning to training and competition, as a second blow to the head can result in a much more serious injury. Recurrent head injury can result in chronic brain damage – a condition seen in up to eighty per cent of professional boxers.

Skull Fracture

A skull fracture may be caused by a heavy blow to the head, especially on impact with a

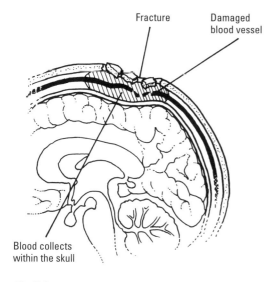

Fracture   Damaged blood vessel

Blood collects within the skull

Skull fracture.

hard surface. Alternatively, the lower part of the skull may be fractured by landing heavily on the base of the spine or when falling from a height and landing heavily on the feet. Always consider the possibility of a neck injury when the head has been injured. It is essential that skull fractures are identified quickly as there is a risk that fragments of broken bone will penetrate the brain, causing further damage. If there is an open wound of the scalp, use a sterile dressing to control bleeding – this will reduce the risk of infectious organisms entering the wound. Fragments of broken bone can also damage underlying blood vessels, leading to bleeding within the skull.

In the event of a heavy impact to the head, the following features may alert the first aider to the possibility of a skull fracture:

- loss of consciousness after sustaining a heavy impact to the head;

- a bleeding wound of the scalp overlying the fracture site;
- a soft area, deformity or depression in the skull;
- blood or fluid discharging from the mouth, nose or ears indicates the presence of a serious injury.

FIRST AID FOR THE UNCONSCIOUS CASUALTY WITH A SUSPECTED SKULL FRACTURE
1. If the casualty is unconscious, lift the chin and tilt the head back to open the airway *unless you suspect a neck or spinal injury* (*see* page 80).
2. Assess the breathing and circulation – you may have to begin CPR. Send someone to call the emergency services and ask for an ambulance.
3. Place the casualty in the recovery position and allow any blood or fluid coming from the mouth, nose or ears to drain.
4. Control any bleeding from the scalp by applying pressure to the sides of the wound with a sterile cloth or dressing.
5. Monitor the casualty's breathing and pulse rate while you wait for help.

FIRST AID FOR THE CONSCIOUS CASUALTY WITH A SUSPECTED SKULL FRACTURE
1. Lie the casualty down with the head and shoulders slightly raised and send someone to call the emergency services and ask for an ambulance.
2. Monitor the casualty's breathing and circulation while you wait for help – the health of a person with a head injury can deteriorate rapidly and you may have to begin CPR.

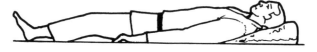

First aid for skull fracture.

3. Allow any blood or fluid coming from the mouth, nose or ears to drain.
4. Control any bleeding from the scalp by applying pressure to the sides of the wound with a sterile cloth or dressing – do not wash the wound or apply any antiseptic or other fluids.

Minor Head Injuries

Clean any superficial cuts and apply a clean dressing to cover the wound. Apply an ice pack wrapped in a towel or cloth to the area to reduce swelling and bruising, and change the ice pack every fifteen to twenty minutes for up to two hours.

Any changes in the level of consciousness of someone who has sustained a head injury, or the development of any of the features listed above will demand urgent medical attention. Following a head injury, however minor, the individual should be monitored closely for several hours afterwards. An injured martial artist should not be allowed to continue training until he is symptom-free for at least one week.

Protective Head Gear

There are many arguments for and against the use of protective head gear in contact sports. Essentially, supporters of the use of padded helmets argue that the fighter is protected from excessively forceful blows to the head. In contrast, detractors of their use argue that fighters are encouraged to hit harder to the head when helmets are worn, thereby negating their usefulness. Furthermore, protective head gear may limit a martial artist's peripheral vision, and helmets with visors are prone to 'steaming up'.

It is advisable that protective head gear should be worn during full-contact sparring, and especially in full-contact competition,

when nervousness can lead to the blunting of reactions, and a reduced level of control. However, the best approach is to teach martial artists to kick and punch to the face *with control* from the earliest stages of training. In this way, by the time a fighter reaches competition level, he has developed the technique and control to execute head kicks and punches without causing injury to an opponent.

Injuries to the Eye

Most martial artists are no strangers to a black eye. Injuries to the eye and its surrounding area are commonly sustained through strikes to the face. The extent of the injury depends on several factors, including the force of the blow and whether the eye is closed at the time of impact. Occasionally, a blow to the eye can cause more serious damage than bruising.

The eye is generally well protected by the eyelid and the bony socket around it. If the eye is closed at the moment of impact, there may be substantial swelling and bruising of the eyelid, but only minimal damage to the eye itself. The characteristic black eye occurs as blood leaks under the skin into the surrounding tissues. As with injuries to other soft tissues, the swelling and bruising can be reduced by applying a cold compress to the area.

The eye itself is made up of several layers, all of which have a role in providing sight. An excessively hard blow may result in detachment, or injury to one or more of these layers, and requires expert attention. It is also possible for the bones around the eyeball, forming the eye socket, to be fractured, resulting in the eye becoming unstable. If this happens, the injured person will complain of double vision.

The following may indicate a serious eye injury:

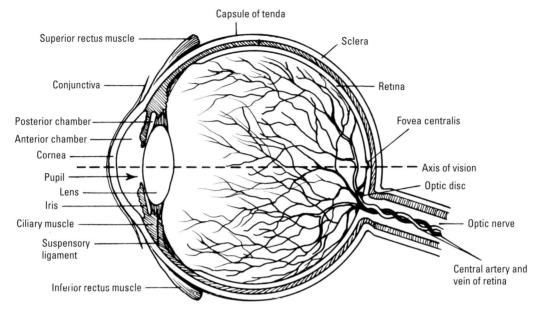

The eye.

- the injured person may complain of blurred or double vision, or loss of vision;
- a severe blow may fracture the bones around the eye, causing the eyeball to take up an abnormal position in the socket; such an injury requires urgent medical attention;
- there may be a wound of the eyelid or the eye itself.

If it is suspected that the casualty has suffered a head injury, concussion, or a neck injury, follow the relevant protocols and seek medical help.

FIRST AID FOR A SUSPECTED FRACTURE OF THE BONES AROUND THE EYE

1. Lie the casualty down with the head and shoulders slightly raised, perhaps resting on your knees.

2. Ask the casualty to close both eyes, keeping the eyes as still as possible.
3. Give the casualty a sterile dressing to hold over the eye.
4. Call the emergency services and ask for an ambulance; the casualty should be transported lying down.

FIRST AID FOR A BLACK EYE

A black eye is the result of blood from damaged tissues collecting under the skin around the eye and eye socket.

1. Apply an ice pack wrapped in a cloth to the bruised area in order to reduce swelling. Change the pack every fifteen to twenty minutes for up to two hours.
2. When the swelling has reduced, a warm compress may help to ease discomfort.

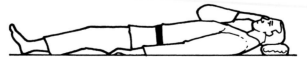

First aid for eye injuries.

A simple black eye should not affect the vision – if the injured person suffers from any blurred or loss of vision, a more serious injury should be suspected.

Contact Lenses

Contact lenses have revolutionized the practice of sports for many people. In general, they can be worn safely for participating in most sports. For contact sports such as the martial arts, soft contact lenses are preferable, as there is less chance of sustaining an abrasion of the cornea while wearing them.

There is a common misconception that a contact lens can become lodged behind the eyeball. In fact, the anatomy of the eyeball and surrounding tissues means that this is impossible. There is, however, a danger that a contact lens can become trapped underneath the eyelid, particularly if a soft lens is torn. In such a situation, it is advisable to attend Casualty, as a thorough examination is required to rule out the possibility of scratches on the cornea, which can become infected. Abrasions of the cornea must be treated correctly as infection can result in permanent damage and loss of vision.

Nose Bleeds

A nose bleed is one of the most common problems in sport. It can occur as a result of minor trauma, or even occur for no apparent reason at all. In younger people, nose bleeds are usually easy to stop, but very occasionally heavy blood loss can be a serious problem. There are also certain medical conditions that predispose people to nose bleeds, such as high blood pressure.

The discharge of blood or fluid from the nose or ears following a head injury can indicate serious damage to the brain, and requires urgent medical attention. The brain and spinal cord are bathed in a clear fluid called cerebrospinal fluid, or CSF, and a

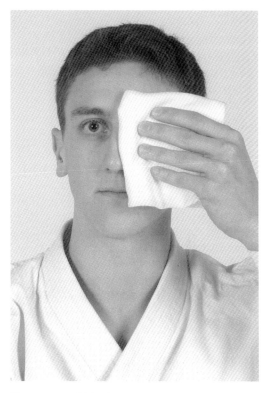

Treatment of black eyes.

severe injury can result in this fluid leaking from the nose or ears.

The central division between the nostrils is known as the septum, and it is from this area at the front of the nose that bleeding usually occurs. The region has a rich blood supply, which is easily damaged. The skin inside the nose is a relatively thin membrane, which is usually protected by nasal mucus. If this mucous membrane becomes dry, the sensitive skin underneath may be exposed, which increases the risk of bleeding.

FIRST AID FOR A NOSE BLEED
1. Sit the casualty down so that he does not fall and sustain further injury.
2. Lean him forward slightly with the head held forward to allow the blood to trickle away from the throat. Do not lie the

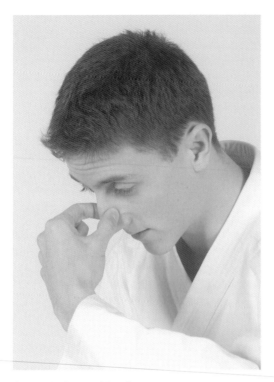

Control of nose bleeds.

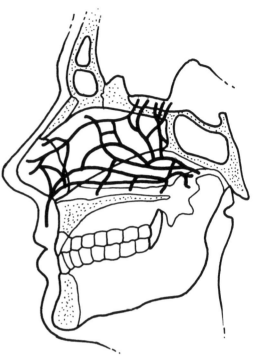

The blood vessels of the nose.

casualty down, as this will increase the risk of inhaling blood.

3. Ask the casualty to pinch the soft part at the front of the nose just below the bridge, with the finger and thumb, in order to compress the bleeding blood vessels.

4. Ask the casualty to breathe through the mouth, and to try not to swallow, speak or sniff, to avoid dislodging the blood clots that will stop the bleeding.

5. After *ten minutes* in this position, check whether the bleeding has stopped – if the nose is still bleeding, pinch the nose below the bridge for *another ten minutes*.

6. A nose bleed that persists for longer than *thirty minutes* requires attention in hospital. Transport the casualty with the head held forward and still applying pressure to the nose.

When the bleeding from the nose has stopped, the martial artist should be advised to rest for several hours, avoiding exercise and the lifting of heavy objects, as well as refraining from blowing the nose.

Nose and Cheekbone Fractures

The bones of the nose and cheek can be fractured by a direct strike to the face, or through being thrown or swept on to a hard surface. The injured martial artist may suffer a nose bleed, and control of heavy bleeding should be a priority (*see* above). The area usually swells considerably, blocking the nasal airways and making breathing through the nose uncomfortable. A broken nose should always be assessed in hospital.

A broken nose or cheekbone may be indicated by the following features:

- the area may become swollen and discoloured, and bruising may appear around the eyes as blood tracks through the soft tissue of the face;
- a fractured nose or cheekbone can be very tender and painful;
- the nose may be more mobile than usual;
- the nose may be displaced to one side;
- the bones of the nose may be visible through a wound (but this is rare).

FIRST AID FOR A SUSPECTED NOSE OR CHEEKBONE FRACTURE

1. Apply an ice pack wrapped in a towel or cloth to the area in order to reduce swelling.
2. Control any bleeding from the nose with pressure on either side of the lower nose (*see* above).
3. Arrange for the casualty to be taken to hospital.

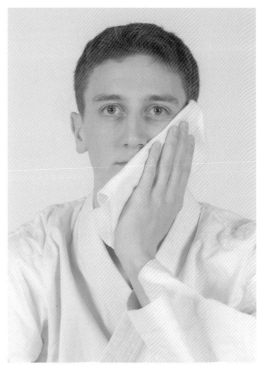

Nose and cheekbone fractures.

A fractured nose will require the attention of a doctor, who will decide whether or not it is necessary to reduce or realign the fracture. Usually it is only possible to treat a fracture before the swelling has arisen; if this has not been feasible, the casualty will have to wait several days for the swelling to ease. It is therefore essential to seek medical attention quickly. It is *not* advisable to attempt to manipulate any displaced bones without expert advice, as this may provoke bleeding. The structure of the nose is made up of both bone and cartilage. As cartilage is less rigid than bone, a fracture can result in the nose becoming highly mobile. If the broken bones are not re-set correctly, the central division, or septum, of the nose may remain deviated, which will alter the flow of air through the nose.

Any cuts in the area will require medical attention for thorough cleaning, to avoid tattooing with dirt.

Injuries to the Mouth, Lips and Teeth

The mouth and lips are commonly cut by strikes to the area, and in some circumstances can bleed heavily. The lining of the mouth may be cut against a sharp tooth, and the lips tend to bleed relatively easily. An unexpected blow may cause a martial artist to bite his own tongue. First aid requires particular attention to prevent blood being swallowed or inhaled.

FIRST AID FOR BLEEDING FROM THE MOUTH

1. Sit the casualty down with the head held slightly forward to allow the blood to

drain away from the mouth – tell the injured person to try not to swallow any blood.

2. The first priority is to control any bleeding – apply a clean dressing to the bleeding area and ask the casualty to apply pressure with the finger and thumb.
3. If the bleeding is from within the mouth, place a dressing over the area and apply pressure from the outside.
4. Replace the dressing if it becomes saturated with blood, and continue to apply pressure.

When the bleeding has stopped, a cold compress or ice pack wrapped in a towel will reduce swelling. Sucking ice cubes can reduce swelling of the tongue. Keeping cuts to the lips moist with a lip balm can promote healing. The casualty should be advised to avoid hot drinks for the next day.

Heavy bleeding for more than thirty

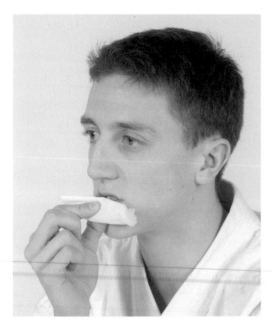

Control of bleeding lips.

minutes, or a particularly large wound, will require professional medical attention.

Knocked-Out Teeth

Many of the injuries that result in the loss of teeth or in a tooth being chipped can be prevented by wearing a well-fitted gum shield when sparring. When a tooth is knocked out, there is a danger that it might be inhaled – if you suspect that this has happened, medical help must be sought urgently. It is also important to realize that an injury that is severe enough to cause a tooth to be knocked out may also be severe enough to damage the jaw.

When dealing with knocked-out teeth, it is essential to act quickly – the earlier a tooth can be replanted in the gum, the greater the chance that it will remain healthy. A dislodged adult tooth should be replaced as soon as possible – there is no need to replace a child's milk tooth.

FIRST AID FOR KNOCKED-OUT TEETH
1. If the tooth socket is bleeding, place a gauze pad thick enough to stop the teeth meeting into the socket – roll it up if necessary.
2. Ask someone to look for the dislodged tooth.
3. Do not wash the tooth as this may damage the living tissue within it. Place the tooth back into its socket and keep it in position by placing a pad or dressing between the upper and lower teeth.
4. If the tooth cannot be replaced in the mouth, keep it in milk or water.
5. Seek the attention of a dentist as soon as possible, or send the casualty to hospital.

Injuries to the Lower Jaw

A heavy, direct blow to the jaw can fracture the jaw bone or mandible. A blow to one side of the jaw can cause a fracture on the opposite side, and a heavy fall on to the chin can result in a fracture of both sides of the mandible.

The jaw is also susceptible to dislocation, especially when a martial artist is struck on the chin while the mouth is open.

The following features indicate some kind of jaw injury:

- pain or nausea on talking or moving the jaw;
- dribbling from one or both sides of the mouth;
- swelling and bruising of the jaw – the area may be tender to the touch;
- a bleeding wound or bruising inside the mouth;
- a severe injury may cause breathing difficulty – monitor the casualty for any signs of distress;
- a jaw injury may accompany a knocked-out tooth.

FIRST AID FOR JAW INJURIES

1. Sit the casualty down with the head held forward to allow any blood or saliva to drain away.
2. If the injured martial artist vomits, support the jaw and head, then gently clean any debris from the mouth so that it cannot be inhaled.
3. Ask the casualty to support the jaw with a soft pad or folded towel – do not bandage or tie the jaw in place, because of the risk of breathing difficulties.
4. Transport the casualty to hospital, keeping the jaw supported.

Injuries of the Throat

The throat can be injured by a direct strike, and also when practising choke holds. Techniques to this vulnerable area must be practised with the utmost caution, as injury

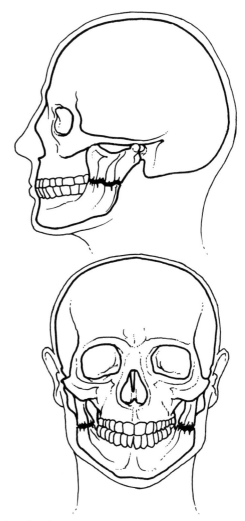

Jaw fracture.

to the throat can be a medical emergency if the airway becomes obstructed. Damage to the throat should always be considered when there has been a neck injury, as trauma to this area is easily missed.

The structure of the throat is maintained by a cartilage skeleton known as the larynx (containing the voice box) and trachea. As cartilage is less strong than bone, the area is particularly vulnerable to compression injuries and fractures.

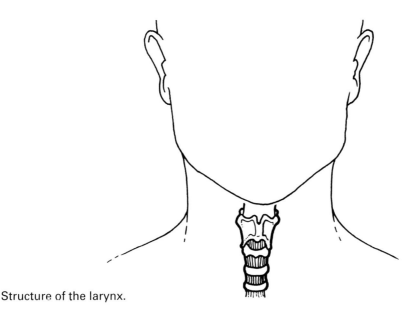

Structure of the larynx.

One function of the larynx and trachea is to carry air to the lungs, and damage to this area can severely obstruct the airway. Any change in the quality of an injured martial artist's voice, or in the sound of his breathing, should be taken as a sign of serious injury.

A blow to the throat may not cause any immediate signs of damage. As with any soft tissue injury, the throat may begin to swell slowly. Over a period of time, breathing will become difficult and this requires immediate medical attention.

Alternatively, the following signs may be immediately apparent and require urgent medical attention:

- sudden difficulty in breathing, with rapid, shallow breaths;
- the casualty's conscious level may start to deteriorate and the injured fighter may collapse;
- if the airway is severely obstructed, the casualty may begin to turn a blue-grey colour, indicating that he is not receiving enough oxygen;
- the casualty, if conscious, may have a hoarse voice or be unable to speak;
- there may be a harsh rasping noise on breathing, known as 'stridor'.

FIRST AID FOR THROAT INJURY
1. Try to remain calm – a distressed casualty needs to be reassured by a calm first aider.
2. Remove any restrictive clothing or jewellery from around the neck.
3. If the martial artist has collapsed, open and assess the airway, then check breathing and circulation. If the casualty is breathing, place him into the recovery position. If the casualty is not breathing, be ready to begin resuscitation. Send someone to call the emergency services and ask for an ambulance while you wait with the casualty.
4. If the casualty is conscious, lie him on the floor with the shoulders raised and help him to remain calm.
5. Keep the casualty's airway open and monitor breathing and pulse rate while you wait for help.

8 Upper Limb Injuries

Dislocated Joints

The Shoulder

The shoulder can be dislocated by an excessively forceful arm lock, and also as a result of being thrown directly on to the shoulder. A martial artist who lands on an outstretched arm is also at risk of suffering a dislocation. Certain people are particularly susceptible to shoulder dislocation, especially if such an injury has been sustained before. The shoulder can be dislocated in any direction, but it is most common for the upper arm to move forwards, out of the socket this is known as an *anterior dislocation*.

The shoulder can also be dislocated when a person suffers a seizure, for example due to epilepsy, as the muscles around the shoulder contract in an uncoordinated manner, pulling the joint out of the socket. The joint formed where the clavicle (collar bone) joins the shoulder can also be dislocated, usually as a result of falling on to the point of the shoulder.

The shoulder is described as a ball and socket joint – the end of the upper arm bone, or humerus, has a spherical shape which inserts into a hollow in the shoulder. This arrangement allows rotational movement but makes it susceptible to

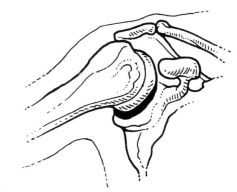

The shoulder joint.

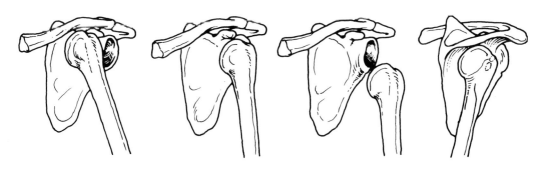

Shoulder dislocations.

dislocation. The joint is surrounded by a capsule and supported by strong ligaments.

The following features are indicators of a dislocated shoulder:

- a lot of pain;
- loss of the normal outline of the shoulder;
- inability to move the arm, and to hold it up without the support of the other arm;
- a numbness to the outer aspect of the arm, as the nerve supplying this area becomes compressed.

FIRST AID FOR A DISLOCATED SHOULDER
1. Ask the casualty to sit down, and place the injured arm across the body. Try to find the position that causes least pain.
2. Pass the point of a triangular bandage through the space between the elbow and arm, and pull it across to the opposite shoulder. If possible, place a soft pad, for example, a folded towel or cloth, between the arm and chest.
3. Fold the opposite point of the bandage over to the injured side. Tie a knot over the shoulder close to the base of the neck to support the injured arm, so that the casualty does not have to bear the weight.
4. Fold the point of the bandage at the elbow forwards, and secure it in place with a safety pin, taking care not to catch the skin underneath.
5. Transport the casualty to hospital, keeping the arm supported and as comfortable as possible.

When the shoulder is dislocated, the strong ligaments supporting the joint may be stretched or damaged. A martial artist who has suffered a dislocation may be susceptible to a similar injury in the future. In some people, an operation to shorten the ligaments may be advised in order to strengthen

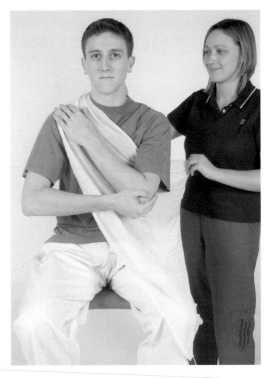

Sling for shoulder dislocation.

the joint. Even if surgery is not advised, it is essential to follow a programme of strengthening exercises to reduce the risk of a second dislocation.

The Fingers and Thumb
The fingers and thumb can be dislocated by falling on to the hand or when blocking a strike, especially if a direct blow to the fingertip is sustained. Finger dislocations are also commonly caused while practising grappling techniques, as fingers are easily caught in clothing.

There are two joints in each finger, and also a joint where the finger joins the hand to form a knuckle. The joints in the fingers are known as hinge joints – they can swing as if on hinges. The joints connecting the finger to the hand are ellipsoid joints – each surface is relatively flat and smooth. These joints are

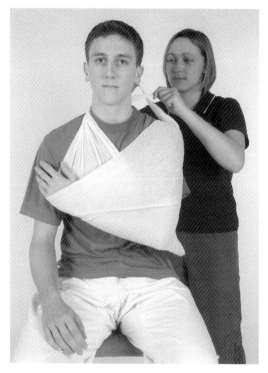

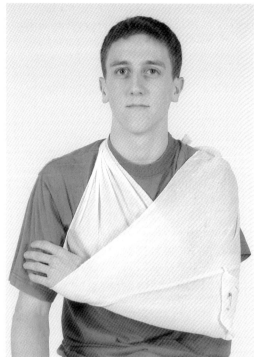

surrounded by capsules and supported by ligaments. The thumb has only one hinge joint and is connected to the hand by what is known as a saddle joint, because of its shape. These joints are held in place by ligaments that are attached to the bones on either side of the joint. A dislocation may indicate that there has been significant damage to these ligaments.

Thumb or finger dislocation may be identified by the following features:

* considerable pain;
* distortion of the normal appearance of the fingers or thumb joints due to displacement of the bones;
* the injured area may be red and can swell very rapidly – try to remove any rings or restrictive clothing from the wrist and hands as soon as possible.

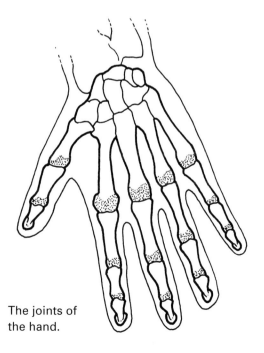

The joints of the hand.

FIRST AID FOR DISLOCATED FINGERS

1. Protect the injured area by wrapping the hand in soft material, then support the arm in an elevated position to reduce swelling.
2. Ask the casualty to support the arm by placing it across the chest with the hand higher than the elbow.
3. Place a triangular bandage over the arm with the longest side running along the injured arm.
4. Fold the bandage under the arm, supporting the injured arm while you work. Pass the lower end of the bandage around the back of the casualty.
5. Tie a knot with the opposite end over the shoulder on the uninjured side. Finally, fold the point of the bandage at the elbow forwards and secure it in place with a safety pin, taking care not to catch the skin underneath.
6. Transport the casualty to hospital with the arm elevated.

It is not recommended to manipulate a dislocated joint back into place, as this may further damage the muscles, nerves or blood supply in the area. After the dislocation has been treated in hospital, the standard regimen of rest, ice and compression will reduce swelling. Later, when the pain has subsided, it is possible to begin gently exercising the joints.

Once a martial artist has sustained a dislocation of a joint in the finger, he may worry that the same thing will happen again, which can lead to a loss of confidence. The risk of repeating such an injury can be

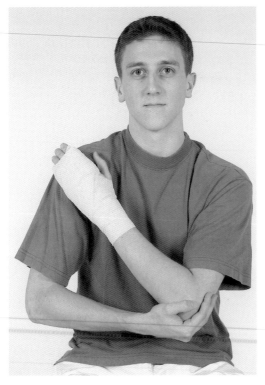
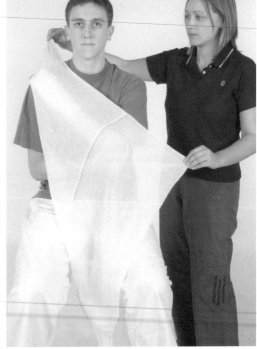

Sling for hand injuries.

reduced by taping the injured finger to an adjacent finger. This technique, known as 'neighbour-strapping', will provide additional support to the previously dislocated joint.

Fractures

Bone is made up of several different layers of material. The inner core comprises a meshwork, which is the bone marrow. Surrounding this core are sheets of strong, dense, but pliable material that give bones both strength and flexibility. Bone is a living tissue, constantly undergoing change and remodelling. It is therefore essential that the blood supply to a bone remains intact.

Fractures or breaks in bones can be sustained through both direct and indirect

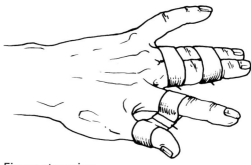

Finger strapping.

forces. A direct force, sufficient to break a bone, might be sustained when a martial artist is thrown on to a hard surface. Indirect forces, especially twisting forces, can also cause cracks in the bone structure. When dealing with fractures, that the first priority is still to control any bleeding. After that, the

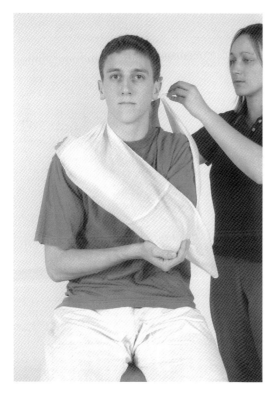

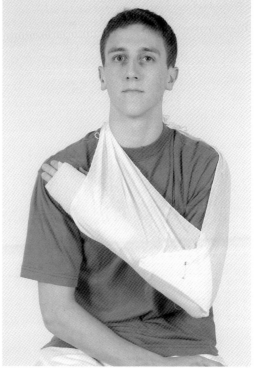

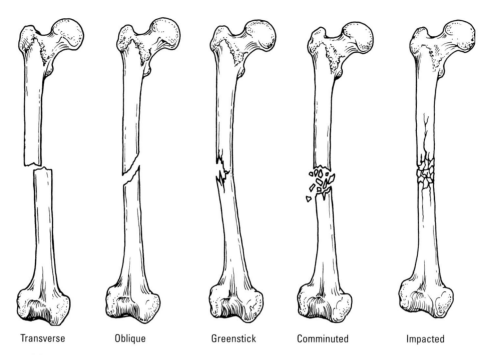

| Transverse | Oblique | Greenstick | Comminuted | Impacted |

Types of fracture.

next priority is to immobilize the limb. This will help to reduce the pain of a fracture, and will also prevent further damage to nearby nerves and arteries.

The term 'fracture' describes the situation in which there is a loss of continuity in the outer layer, or cortex, of a bone. There are several types of fracture – a bone may break cleanly or shatter into several pieces. When a fracture causes a bone to perforate the over-lying skin, it is known as an *open fracture*, and it can be accompanied by severe bleeding. In a *closed fracture* both ends of the bones remain within the skin; this can also cause bleeding, but this time it is internal.

The Collar Bone

The collar bone (or clavicle) connects the shoulder to the breastbone, and provides stability to the arm and shoulder girdle. This bone transmits forces from the shoulder to the trunk. The collar bone is more commonly broken by a direct force – a martial artist who falls with the arms outstretched is particularly vulnerable. The most common site for a break to occur is in the middle section of the clavicle.

The following features may indicate a fracture of the collar bone:

- a lot of pain in the area, which intensifies when trying to move the injured arm;
- the casualty may try to find the least painful position for the arm – this is often supporting the arm at the elbow with the head leaning towards the injured side;
- the most tender area will often be over the middle of the clavicle, halfway between the shoulder and sternum (breastbone);
- loss of the normal outline of the shoulder, as the muscles pull on the two separated fragments of bone.

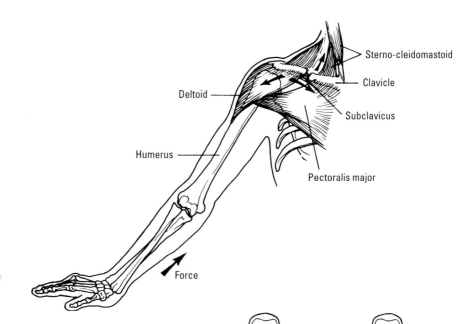

Sterno-cleidomastoid

Clavicle

Deltoid

Subclavicus

Humerus

Pectoralis major

Force

Fracture of the collar bone.

FIRST AID FOR A FRACTURED COLLAR BONE

1. The first priority is to control any heavy bleeding with direct pressure over the wound.
2. Ask the casualty to sit down. Try to find the position that causes least pain – usually this is to place the injured arm across the chest and support it at the elbow.
3. Place a triangular bandage over the arm, with the longest side running along the injured arm.
4. Fold the bandage under the injured arm, supporting it while you work, in order to reduce the pain.
5. Pass the lower end of the bandage around the back of the casualty, then tie a knot with the opposite end over the uninjured shoulder. Supporting the arm will reduce the pain – it may be necessary to tie a bandage around the arm and chest to provide further support.
6. Transport the casualty to hospital with the arm elevated.

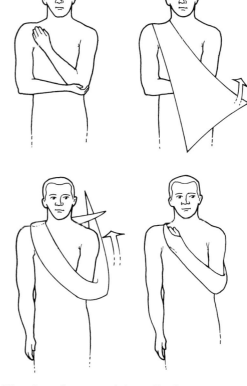

Sling for a fracture of the collar bone.

101

The Upper Arm

The upper arm (or humerus) is relatively strong, and fractures of this bone are rare in young, healthy people. It can be broken by a direct strike, but is more often fractured as the result of a fall. The area near the elbow is particularly susceptible to injury when falling on to an outstretched arm – this type of fracture is more commonly seen in children. It is also possible for a fracture to be caused by chronic over-use, but this is more often seen in sports that involve repetitive throwing movements.

A martial artist may not realize that the bone of the upper arm has been fractured, because the arm may remain fairly stable, as a result of the action of the large muscles that pull along the line of the upper arm.

A fracture of the humerus close to the elbow requires urgent immobilization and medical attention. Any small pieces of shattered bone are a threat to the arteries and nerves that pass close to the elbow joint. The status of the arteries and nerves beyond a fracture of the upper arm may be monitored by checking the radial pulse, and assessing the sensation in the casualty's fingers at regular intervals.

A fracture of the upper arm (humerus) may be indicated by the following features:

- constant pain, worsened by moving the arm;
- the arm will be tender to the touch;
- swelling of the damaged tissue and slow development of bruising;
- if the elbow has been damaged, there may be an inability to straighten the arm.

FIRST AID FOR AN UPPER ARM FRACTURE

1. The first priority is to immobilize the arm.
2. Ask the casualty to sit down. Place the injured arm across the chest if it is possible to bend the elbow. Try to find the position that causes least pain. If possible, ask the casualty to support the arm.
3. Pass the point of a triangular bandage through the space between the elbow and arm, and pull it across to the opposite shoulder. Place a soft pad, for example, a folded towel or cloth, between the arm and chest.
4. Fold the opposite point of the bandage over to the injured side and tie a knot over the shoulder close to the base of the neck.
5. Fold the point of the bandage at the elbow forwards, and secure it in place with a safety pin.
6. If a second triangular bandage is available, fold the point to touch the base of the triangle. Fold the bandage in half again, and use this broad-fold bandage to secure the arm by tying it around the chest.
7. Transport the casualty to hospital, keeping them seated as much as possible.

If the elbow cannot be bent, lay the injured martial artist on the floor, and place soft padding around the injured arm. Do not try to force the arm to bend as this may cause damage to nearby arteries and nerves. Call the emergency services and ask for an ambulance.

The Forearm and Wrist

The bones of the forearm may be fractured by a heavy strike, or while blocking an attack. A fracture in this location may cause pieces of broken bone to penetrate the skin, producing an open fracture. Falling on to an outstretched hand may cause a characteristic break in the wrist.

The wrist is very rarely dislocated, but sprains of this joint are commonly sustained through wrist locks and falls. Injuries of the wrist are more common in children.

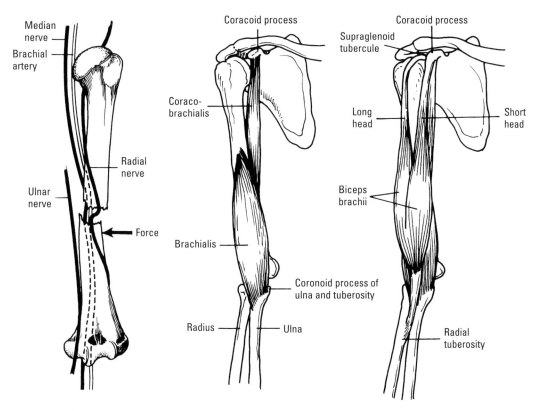

Fracture of the humerus. The muscles of the upper arm.

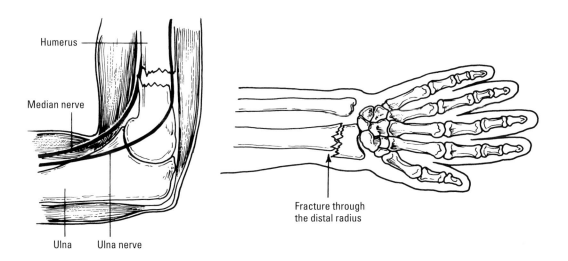

Fracture of lower humerus.   Wrist fracture.

A fractured forearm or wrist may be indicated by the following features:

- pain in the area, and a tenderness to the touch;
- an open wound, formed by the ends of the broken bone piercing the skin;
- rapid swelling, and the development of bruising;
- an alteration in the normal outline of the wrist, known as a 'dinner-fork' deformity.

FIRST AID FOR WRIST FRACTURES
1. The first priority is to immobilize the arm, to prevent further damage.
2. Ask the casualty to sit down. Support the injured arm across the casualty's chest, or lay it across the lap on some soft padding. If there is an open wound, cover it with a clean pad and apply gentle pressure to control any bleeding – do not press directly on to the end of any fractured bones.
3. Pass the point of a triangular bandage through the gap between the elbow and arm, then pull it across to the opposite shoulder.

4. Fold the opposite point of the bandage over to the injured side and tie a knot over the shoulder.
5. Fold the point of the bandage at the elbow forwards and secure it with tape or a pin. Transport the casualty to hospital, keeping him seated whenever possible.

The Hand
The bones of the hand can be fractured as a result of striking both with a fist and with an open hand. Beginners should be taught to form a fist correctly, never placing the thumb inside the fingers. Bones can also be fractured by a fall on to an outstretched hand. Punching can result in compression or stress fractures.

It is essential that any suspected fracture of the hand is X-rayed promptly. When the scaphoid (one of the bones in the palm of the hand) is fractured, there is a possibility that the blood supply to part of the bone may be compromised. If this situation is not treated correctly, part of the bone may die, leading to pain and arthritis. A fracture of the scaphoid bone is characterized by pain between the two tendons at the base of the

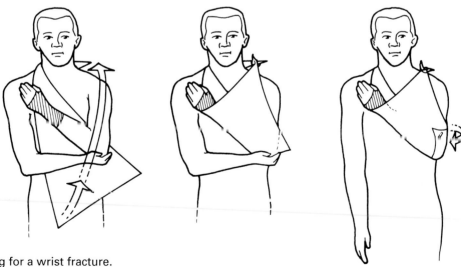

Sling for a wrist fracture.

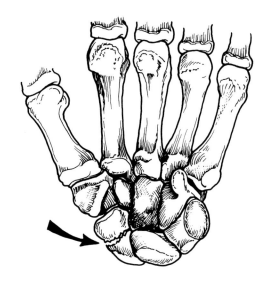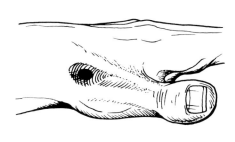

Scaphoid fracture and tenderness in the 'anatomical snuff box'.

thumb – an area known as the 'anatomical snuff box'. The treatment involves plaster casting for several weeks, to ensure correct healing.

Particular areas in the hand are more prone to fracture than others. One of these fractures has earned the name of the 'boxer's fracture' or the 'Saturday-night fracture', because of the frequency with which it is seen in hospitals after Saturday-night brawls.

A fracture of the hand may be indicated by the following features:

- considerable pain;
- tenderness to the touch and rapid swelling – this is one of the reasons why rings and other tight jewellery should never be worn when training in martial arts;
- distortion of the normal outline of the fingers as fragments of bone rotate or are displaced.

FIRST AID FOR FRACTURES OF THE HAND
The procedure is the same as for dislocations of the fingers.

1. Protect the injured area by wrapping the hand in soft material, then support the arm in an elevated position to reduce swelling.
2. Ask the casualty to support the arm by placing it across the chest with the hand higher than the elbow (see the pictures on page 98).
3. Place a triangular bandage over the arm with the longest side running along the injured arm.
4. Fold the bandage under the arm, supporting the injured arm while you work.
5. Pass the lower end of the bandage around the back of the casualty. Then tie a knot with the opposite end over the shoulder on the uninjured side.
6. Transport the casualty to hospital with the arm elevated.

The hand is a common site of injury and it is essential that any hand injury is assessed and managed effectively, in order to avoid permanent loss of function. A systematic approach to hand trauma will identify which

105

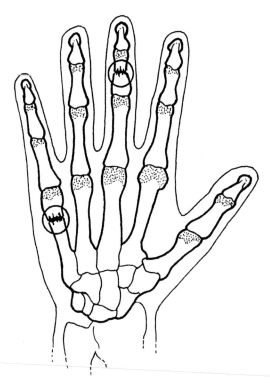

Common sites of fracture.

structures within the hand are damaged, and whether expert help is required. Each of the components of the hand should be considered in turn:

- skin;
- muscles;
- tendons;
- blood vessels;
- nerves;
- bones.

When a cut to the hand has been sustained, consider whether deeper structures have been damaged. Injury to arteries will be evident from profuse bleeding. Damage to nerves will result in loss of sensation, or movement of the fingers. Similarly, when a tendon is cut or ruptured, the injured person

will be unable to bend the fingers. A bony injury may be suspected when the fingers appear out of shape, and when there is prolonged tenderness of a bony area. Hand injuries tend to swell quickly, which can lead to permanent stiffness and reduced function. For this reason an injured hand should be elevated in a sling as quickly as possible, and assessed in hospital.

Sprains

The joints of the body are held together by tough bands known as ligaments, which attach one bone to another, and act across a joint. A sprain is the result of injury to these ligaments. Sprains are caused by excessive movement of a joint, which forces it to move further than its normal range of motion.

The Shoulder
The ligaments surrounding the shoulder have an important role in stabilizing the joint and the collar bone. The shoulder may be sprained as a result of movement outside the normal range, such as an excessively forceful arm lock, or during a fall on to the shoulder. Such an injury may also damage the capsule surrounding the joint, or the tendons of nearby muscles.

A sprained shoulder will share some of the features of a dislocated joint, but without any distortion of the normal appearance. The joint will be painful, especially on movement, and the area may begin to swell over several hours.

FIRST AID FOR A SPRAINED SHOULDER
The principles of treating any soft-tissue injury can be applied to the shoulder joint:

P – Protect the injured joint from further damage.
R – Rest the injured shoulder for several days.

I – Ice the area or apply a cold compress.

C – Compress the injured area. This principle can be difficult to apply to the shoulder, however, elasticated support bandages can be obtained.

E – Elevate the injured joint in a sling or on a pillow when resting.

The rotator cuff is the group of muscles which act around the shoulder joint, to stabilize it, and allow its wide range of movement. These muscles act whenever a punch is thrown, or the arms are raised above the head. As a result, the rotator cuff is placed under a great deal of stress through martial arts training. Injuries are more common as people get older, but small tears in the muscles are relatively common. It is also quite common for older people to suffer complete tears of these muscles, which may require surgical treatment.

A martial artist who suffers an injury to the rotator cuff may find it difficult to lift the arm from the side of the body, or may have limited movement of the shoulder. These features are likely to be due to weakness of the muscles, or swelling as a result of trauma.

Injuries to the rotator cuff should be managed using the standard treatment of rest, ice, compression. Once the symptoms resolve, it is important to follow a regimen of strengthening exercises, and the advice of a physiotherapist should be sought. In occasional circumstances, steroid injections or surgery may be required to resolve the symptoms of pain and weakness.

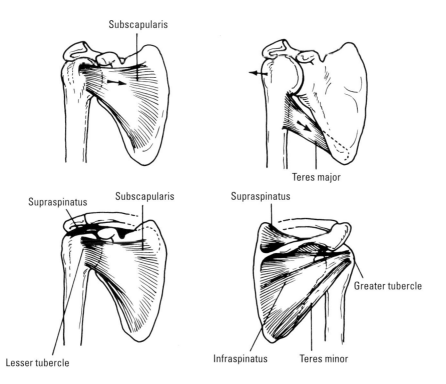

The rotator cuff.

The Wrist

The wrist is one of the most commonly injured joints. It is easy to understand why, when the anatomy of the joint is considered. The wrist joint is made up of the two forearm bones – the radius and ulna – which join eight bones within the palm of the hand. Many ligaments join these bones together and act to stabilize the joint, and they all come under a great deal of stress as the wrist is capable of a wide range of movement. Several martial arts take advantage of this anatomical arrangement, through the teaching of wrist-locking techniques. The pain felt when a wrist lock is applied correctly arises as a result of tension placed on the tendons and ligaments acting within the joint. Wrist locks should be practised with caution, as it is easy to overestimate how much force an opponent's wrist can withstand.

A sprained wrist is a relatively common injury, and can be sustained by falling on to an outstretched hand. Such an injury may also result in a fracture of the wrist.

Excessive bending of the wrist both upwards and downwards, which can occur when wrist locks are applied, can cause damage to the ligaments supporting the wrist, resulting in a painful injury.

A sprained wrist will display the following features:

- pain that increases on moving the joint;
- tenderness to the touch over the wrist joint;
- the injured area may become hot, red and swollen.

FIRST AID FOR A SPRAINED WRIST

The principles of treating any soft-tissue injury can be applied to the wrist joints:

P – Protect the injured limb from further damage.
R – Rest the injured wrist for several days.
I – Ice the area or apply a cold compress.
C – Compress the injured area.
E – Elevate the injured wrist in a sling or on a pillow when resting.

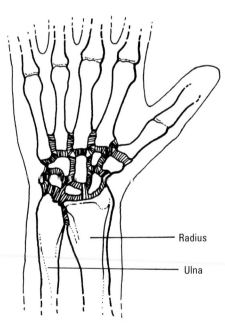

Radius

Ulna

The wrist joint.

After resting the wrist until it is completely pain-free, it will be possible to begin activity again gradually. The injured joint may be more susceptible to injury, and it is recommended to seek advice regarding progressive exercise regimes to strengthen the joint. It is also advisable to use elasticated wrist supports in the early stages of training after such an injury.

Fingers and Thumbs

The joints of the hand may be sprained as a result of a strike or block, or any activity that causes excessive bending at a joint. Such injuries must be treated carefully to ensure that the full range of movement of the joint is regained.

If a finger or thumb is sprained, the area may swell quickly, obscuring the normal appearance of the joint, and the joint will be painful and tender to the touch. A severe injury may result in the joint becoming unstable, as the ligament may be ruptured.

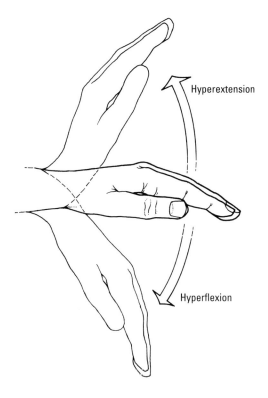

Hyperflexion and hyperextension of the wrist.

FIRST AID FOR FINGER AND THUMB SPRAINS

A minor sprain injury of the joints of the hand can be treated following the principles for any soft-tissue injury:

P – Protect
R – Rest
I – Ice
C – Compress
E – Elevate

Severe pain or instability of a joint should alert you to the possibility of more serious injury. All such injuries should be assessed in hospital as a further precaution, for damage to the bone or nearby nerves. It may also be necessary to begin moving the injured joint at an early stage to prevent any loss of mobility.

9 The Chest and Abdomen

Fractured Ribs

The ribcage comprises twelve pairs of ribs, which protect the organs of the chest – the lungs, heart and major arteries and veins.

The lungs are enclosed within an airtight space – the gap between the lungs and the chest wall – called the pleural cavity. They are made up of highly elastic tissues and there is, therefore, a natural tendency for them to collapse. The lungs are prevented from collapsing by the negative pressure that exists within the pleural space. A fractured rib-end can puncture this space, causing the lung to collapse, as the negative pressure is lost. A collapsed lung causes difficulty breathing because only one functioning lung remains to exchange oxygen for carbon dioxide; taking deep breaths can become very painful.

A fracture of the ribs can be caused by a direct blow, or can occur as a result of a crushing injury. If the chest wall is penetrated by a sharp object, air may be drawn into the chest with every breath the casualty takes. This is a medical emergency, and needs urgent action to stabilize the casualty and to ensure rapid medical attention. Asthmatics are also at risk of suffering from a collapsed lung, and this can happen without any trauma to the chest.

A fractured rib may cause the following features in the injured martial artist:

* considerable pain, which is worse when breathing in;

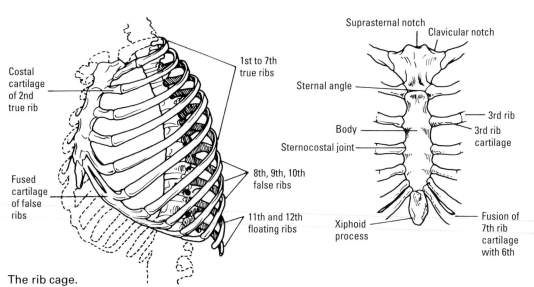

The rib cage.

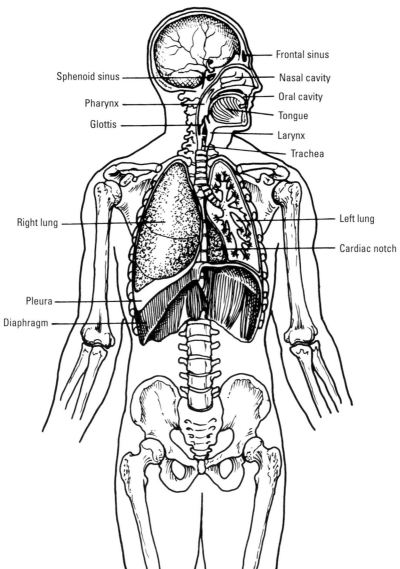

Sphenoid sinus

Pharynx

Glottis

Frontal sinus

Nasal cavity

Oral cavity

Tongue

Larynx

Trachea

Right lung

Left lung

Cardiac notch

Pleura

Diaphragm

The lungs.

- a tendency to take short, shallow breaths in an attempt to avoid the pain;
- extreme tenderness in the area of the fracture;
- distortion in the shape of the chest wall at the site of the broken rib;
- there may be an open wound over the fracture – this is a medical emergency.

FIRST AID FOR FRACTURED RIBS WITHOUT AN OPEN WOUND
1. Ask the injured martial artist to sit down and make him as comfortable as possible.
2. Observe the casualty. If he is struggling to breathe, call the emergency services and ask for an ambulance, or take him

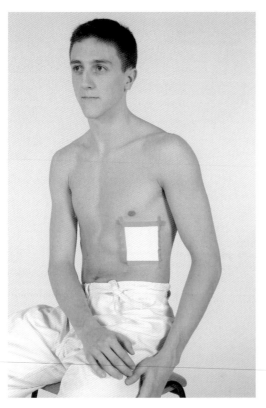

Dressing for rib fracture with an open wound.

safety pin, ensuring that you do not catch the skin underneath.

4. Monitor the casualty's breathing while you take him to hospital.

FIRST AID FOR FRACTURES WITH AN OPEN WOUND

1. Sit the casualty down and lean him towards the side of the injury. Immediately cover any open wound with the palm of the casualty's hand, or use your own hand until a dressing is available.

2. Place a clean square dressing over the wound, and secure the dressing with tape on three sides. *Do not stick down the fourth side of the square.* This will allow air to leave the chest as the casualty breathes out, but will prevent air from entering the chest.

3. Call the emergency services and ask for an ambulance.

4. Support the arm on the side of the wound with a sling. Ask the casualty to place the arm across the chest, with the hand higher than the elbow. Place a triangular bandage over the arm with the longest side running along the top of the arm. Fold the bandage under the arm. Pass the lower end of the bandage around the back of the casualty. Then tie a knot with the opposite end over the shoulder on the side of the injury.

5. Observe the casualty closely until the ambulance arrives – if breathing becomes difficult, place the casualty into the recovery position.

to hospital immediately. Do not wait until the injured person turns blue.

3. If the casualty can talk normally, and there are no open wounds, place the arm on the side of the injury in an arm sling (*see* the pictures on page 98). Place the arm on the injured side across the body; try to find the position that causes least pain. Pass the point of a triangular bandage through the space between the elbow and arm, and pull it across to the opposite shoulder. Fold the opposite point of the bandage over the injured side, and tie a knot over the shoulder close to the base of the neck. Fold the point of the bandage at the elbow forwards, and secure it in place with a

Injuries of the ribs, including fractures and bruises, are very common. In most cases, the ribs are not displaced, and the mainstay of treatment is rest for six to eight weeks. It can take a relatively long time for rib fractures to heal, as the ribcage is constantly moving with each breath. It is very difficult to distin-

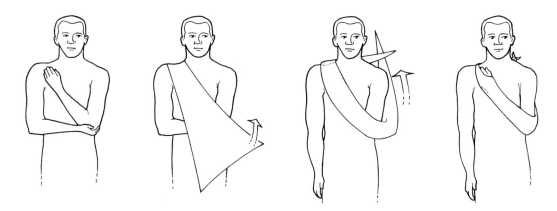

Elevation sling for a rib fracture with an open wound.

guish a rib fracture from a simple bruise, as both can be very painful. It is therefore essential that all suspected fractures are X-rayed promptly. Occasionally, a fractured rib causes damage to the underlying lung, and this is a situation which can be life-threatening.

It is advisable for female martial artists to wear a chest guard whenever participating in contact activities, and especially in the competitive arena.

The Abdomen

Anatomically, the abdomen is the area between the thorax (chest) and the pelvis. It is separated from the thorax by the diaphragm, but is continuous with the pelvis. The abdomen contains the majority of the digestive organs – the stomach, small and large intestines, the liver, pancreas, gall bladder and also the spleen and kidneys. The major blood vessels continue from the chest cavity through the diaphragm and into the abdomen.

Liver and Spleen

The liver performs many important functions, which include the storage of glucose as glycogen, the production of factors which

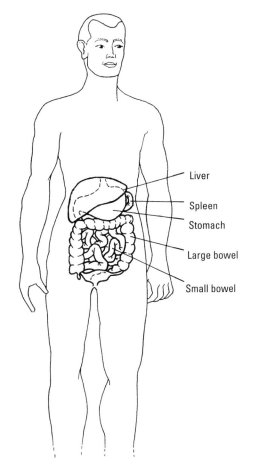

The abdominal organs.

allow the blood to clot, and the processing of proteins from the diet. It is therefore essential for life. The spleen also has several important roles, and is involved in protecting the body from infection. It is possible for a person to survive if the spleen is removed, although one side effect is an increased susceptibility to certain infections.

Although both the liver and spleen are protected by the ribcage, the spleen is the most commonly damaged abdominal organ. It is particularly susceptible when blows are sustained to the left lower chest. It has a tendency to bleed profusely, and such an injury can result in a casualty becoming severely compromised and shocked. Splenic injury requires rapid medical attention. Often, it is difficult to control the bleeding, and the only solution is to remove the spleen surgically in order to prevent the casualty from dying.

It is possible for the liver to be injured by blows to the lower right side of the chest. A fractured rib may result in a laceration of the liver and severe bleeding, but this is less common.

The Kidneys

The kidneys lie at the back of the abdomen and are consequently relatively well protected. Their function is to filter the blood, and thereby control the composition of water and salts within the body. The kidneys are therefore essential organs for the normal function of the body.

It is possible for the kidneys to be damaged by blows to the lower back and also in falls from a height. Injuries to the kidney can be serious, and one feature of serious injury is passing blood in the urine. The kidneys are connected to the bladder by long tubular structures called the ureters. Damage to a kidney, or its ureter, can result in urine leaking into the abdomen, and this requires urgent surgical repair. Less commonly, the bladder may be injured by strikes to the lower abdomen. Blood in the urine should alert you to such an injury. The bladder may also be damaged when the pelvic bones are fractured, but this injury requires significant forces and is most commonly seen in the context of road traffic accidents.

Winding

A person feels winded when struck unexpectedly, without having the opportunity to tense the abdominal muscles. Usually, the situation is quickly resolved by taking several

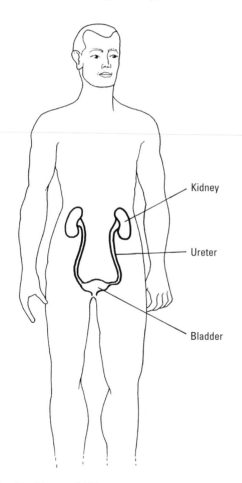

Kidney

Ureter

Bladder

The bladder and kidneys.

deep breaths. Ask the casualty to stand upright and place his hands behind the head – this position stabilizes the shoulders and allows the lungs to be fully expanded with each breath.

The Genitalia

Injuries to the genitalia can be largely prevented by wearing a box, or other protective equipment, when sparring. The importance of groin protectors should not be underestimated, as genital injuries can be extremely serious.

The Urethra

The urethra is the tubular connection from the bladder to the outside, which allows us to urinate. In men, the urethra is long and travels through the penis, whereas in women, the urethra is very short. For this reason, the male urethra is much more prone to injury. It can be damaged by blows between the legs, and also when bones within the pelvis are fractured. Features of urethral injury include passing blood in the urine, inability to pass water, and, in men, blood at the tip of the penis. Such an injury requires urgent attention in hospital.

Torsion of the Testicle

A torsion of the testicle occurs when the testicle becomes twisted within the scrotum, impeding its blood supply. It is most common in young men and may be due to a particular anatomical arrangement that makes certain men more susceptible than others. A testicular torsion can occur as a result of trauma to the area, but is most commonly seen when there has been no injury to the testicle. When torsion occurs, the testicle swells rapidly and is extremely painful. Later the scrotum becomes red, swollen and tender. A suspected testicular torsion should be assessed in hospital as quickly as possible, so that the blood supply can be restored at the earliest opportunity.

10   Lower Limb Injuries

In a healthy person, the bones of the leg can only be broken by considerable forces, such as those generated in road traffic accidents. A fracture of the thigh bone (or femur) is important to recognize because it can cause a significant amount of unseen, or internal, bleeding. However, such an injury is rare in the martial arts. Elderly people are much more prone to a fracture of the femur, as a result of osteoporosis (a process that weakens the bones making them more susceptible to injury).

It is also possible for the femur to be affected by a stress fracture, which occurs as a result of repeated stresses on the bone. This is more commonly associated with endurance events such as marathon running. The pain of a stress fracture is usually more persistent and generalized in nature than the pain of a sudden fracture that occurs as a result of trauma.

The Knee

The knee is a hinge joint formed by the lower end of the femur (thigh bone) and the upper end of the tibia (shin bone). As it is a hinge joint, it is designed to swing forwards and backwards only, in one plane (although the natural movement of the knee includes a limited amount of rotational motion). The knee is held secure by strong ligaments and muscles acting across the joint. Excessive movements, outside of the normal range, can damage these ligaments and muscles.

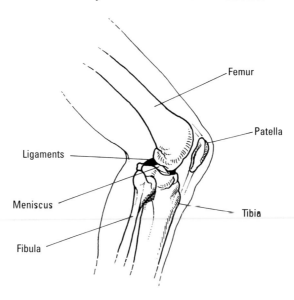

The knee joint.

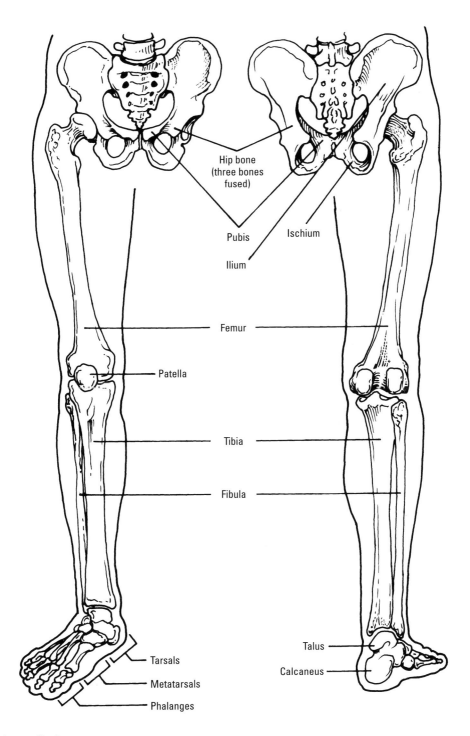

The lower limbs.

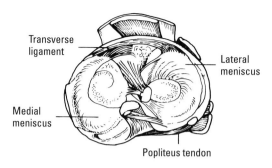

Transverse ligament

Lateral meniscus

Medial meniscus

Popliteus tendon

The menisci.

The knee joint is placed under a considerable amount of strain during the course of a typical training session. Consequently, it is one of the most commonly injured joints. It is also relatively common for the knee to be affected by chronic disorders, such as osteoarthritis, which may be a consequence of long-term wear and tear of the cartilage within the knee joint. Complete dislocations of the knee however, are rarely seen outside the context of high-energy impacts, such as road traffic accidents.

The knee can be damaged by a direct blow, especially to the front of the knee when the leg is straight, or by twisting and turning motions. A common cause of strain on the knee in martial arts is poor technique when moving forwards and backwards in front stance – pointing the toes too far inwards or outwards can place excessive pressure on the ligaments.

Injuries to the Cartilage
A significant number of forces act through the knees during the course of a normal day, and they need to be capable of a wide range of movements. Simply standing up from a chair or climbing a flight of stairs places considerable demands on the joint. Even in an everyday context, the structure of the knee must allow it to cope with all sorts of stresses. Now consider the demands placed on the knee during the course of an average

martial arts training session, which may involve running, jumping and kicking, all done barefoot and on a hard surface. It is easy to see why this particular joint is so commonly injured.

Between the lower surface of the femur and the upper surface of the tibia there are two semi-circular pieces of cartilage, known as the *medial* and *lateral menisci*. The menisci are thought to act as shock absorbers, designed to dissipate some of the force transmitted through the knee when walking or jumping. The surface of this cartilage is smooth, which also aids movement.

The menisci can be torn as a result of a sudden twisting of the knee, while the foot remains stationary on the floor. This can result in part of the torn cartilage becoming trapped within the joint, and preventing the knee from bending – this is known as locking of the joint. Such an injury can be very painful, and can result in a substantial amount of swelling.

Injuries to the Ligaments
Several ligaments act within and across the knee joint, to provide stability. As the knee is a hinge joint, it should move only in one plane. Excessive side-to-side movement is prevented by the collateral ligaments, which attach across the inside and outside of the joint. A blow to the outside of the knee is likely to damage the medial collateral ligament as the knee will bend inwards. Conversely, a blow to the outside of the knee is likely to damage the lateral collateral. It is therefore essential that leg-sweep techniques are aimed well below the knee; indeed, in some competitions, the rules allow sweeps only below the ankle. The medial collateral ligament, on the inside of the knee, is often damaged in association with the medial meniscus.

The anterior and posterior cruciate ligaments are within the knee joint, and act to prevent excessive movement backwards and forwards. These ligaments are essential for the stability of the knee, therefore tearing of the cruciate ligaments can result in the knee becoming highly unstable.

The anterior cruciate is more commonly damaged in sporting injuries. The casualty may even recall a 'popping' noise as the ligament tears. In such an injury, the knee swells very rapidly as the joint fills with blood. This ligament is most likely to be injured as a result of twisting the bent knee, or as a result of over-straightening (hyperextending) the joint.

Both meniscal and ligament injuries may require surgical repair. After such surgery it is essential for the injured martial artist to complete a course of rehabilitative exercises to strengthen the joint. Without this period of rehabilitation, the injured knee would soon suffer from stiffness, and a resulting

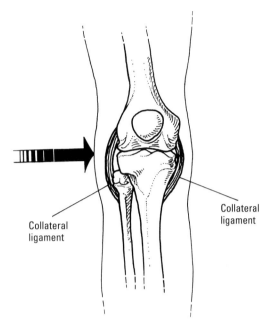

Injury to the collateral ligaments.

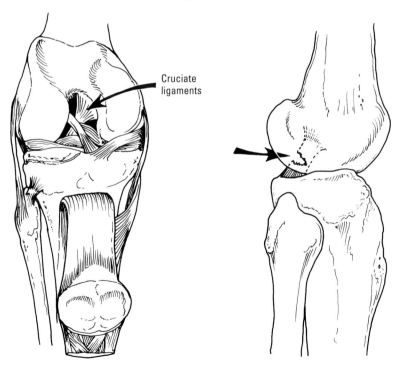

The cruciate ligaments.

loss of function. It can be a long and arduous process for a martial artist to recover his pre-injury level of activity.

An injury to the knee may be indicated by a number of features:

- a torn or strained ligament may cause considerable pain that is localized to the knee joint;
- the knee may swell rapidly and become tender to the touch;
- there may be an inability to bend the knee if it becomes locked and painful – this may be due to a piece of fractured bone or cartilage becoming trapped inside the joint.

FIRST AID FOR KNEE INJURY

1. Ask the casualty to lie down, and place a cushion or soft material under the injured knee. Try to find a position for the knee which causes least pain.
2. Do not try to force the knee to bend, as this may cause further damage to the joint, as well as to nearby blood vessels and nerves.
3. Protect the damaged knee by gently placing soft padding around it, then wrap a bandage around the knee to keep the padding in place. Apply an ice pack to the area and elevate the leg, if the casualty can tolerate this movement.
4. The casualty should be transported to hospital with the leg straight, and not allowed to bear weight on the injured knee. If the casualty is in too much pain to be moved, call for an ambulance, as a stretcher will be required.

The Knee Cap

The knee cap, or patella, can be fractured or dislocated by a direct blow to the front of the knee. This bone is actually a structure within the tendon of the quadriceps muscle, which attaches to the tibia just below the knee. Weakness of the quadriceps increases the risk of dislocating the patella.

If a fighter sustains a dislocation of the patella, he should be taken to hospital to allow a doctor to replace it. It is not advisable to manipulate the knee cap unless you have expert training, as this may cause further damage to the quadriceps tendon, and to other nearby structures. If you suspect a fracture of the patella, follow the principles of P, R, I, C, E – protection, rest, ice, compression and elevation – then transport the casualty to hospital.

After sustaining a dislocated patella, it is advisable to wear an elasticated knee support, to reduce the risk of a recurrence.

Fractures of the Lower Leg

The lower leg comprises two bones: the *tibia* (shin bone), which is strong and thick, and the *fibula*, which is thinner and weaker.

In healthy people, the tibia is usually only broken by strong, direct forces such as those sustained in heavy falls from a height, or road accidents. The tibia is more commonly affected by stress fractures, as a result of repetitive activities on hard surfaces. The thinner fibula is more easily damaged, however, and can be fractured as a result of excessive twisting of the lower leg. If only the fibula is broken, the injury may go unnoticed, and the injured martial artist may continue to walk as normal.

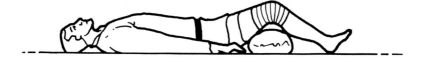

Knee injury.

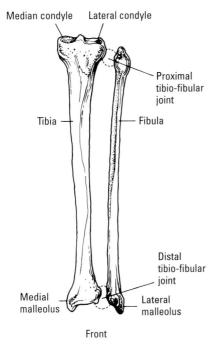

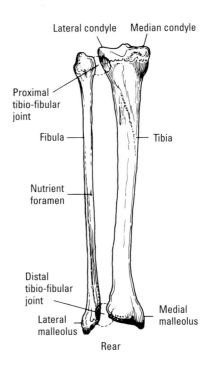

The lower leg.

A broken shin bone may be indicated by the following features:

- pain localized to the lower leg;
- a wound over the site of the fracture or bone penetrating the skin;
- rapid swelling in the area;
- an inability to walk.

FIRST AID FOR FRACTURES OF THE SHIN

1. Help the casualty to lie down. The first priority is to control any bleeding by placing a dressing, and applying pressure over the wound. If the ends of the bone are protruding through the skin, do not press directly on them – apply pressure at the sides of the wound.
2. Do not try to straighten the leg by pulling along the line of the shin bone. This may cause damage to nearby blood vessels and nerves.
3. Send someone to call the emergency services and ask for an ambulance.
4. Place soft padding under the leg and support the broken the ambulance arrives.

Muscle Cramps

The calf muscles are most commonly affected by cramps. A cramp occurs when the muscle fibres contract and come under tension, but do not relax. The exact cause for this is unknown, but, as cramps are more common in hot weather, it is thought that dehydration may be an important factor. The calf muscles are also very active during exercise, and therefore require a substantial supply of blood. Any compromise of the blood vessels to these muscles will reduce the blood flow, and also cause cramping pains.

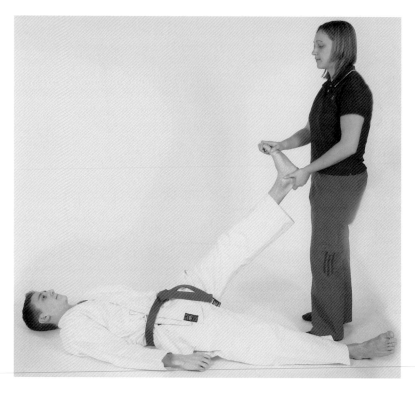

Calf cramps.

A martial artist suffering from calf cramps should be asked to lie on his back. Massaging the muscles will promote blood flow to the area, and gently flexing the ankle will help to reduce the pain, and ease any muscle spasm.

Ankle Sprains

The ankle is a joint formed by the lower end of the shin bone (tibia) and the bones of the foot. It is a highly mobile joint, and must therefore be stabilized by strong ligaments and muscles acting across the joint.

A sprained ankle is a common injury in many sports, and the martial arts are no exception. A sprain is usually caused by excessive twisting of the ankle, which results in injury to the ligaments acting across the sides of the joint (the collateral ligaments). The most commonly affected ligaments are those on the outside of the joint, as the commonest mechanism of injury is 'going over' on the foot – a so-called 'inversion strain'. The risk of sustaining such an injury is increased by training on uneven ground, or torn mats.

It is also possible for the ligaments to be torn if they are subjected to severe over-stretching. Such an injury results in severe pain and rapid swelling of the ankle. A tearing noise may even be heard at the time of injury.

A sprained ankle may cause the following:

- extreme pain, which is usually worse on moving the ankle;
- rapid swelling and bruising, particularly over the inner and outer aspects of the joint;
- an inability to walk, as the ankle may be too painful to bear weight.

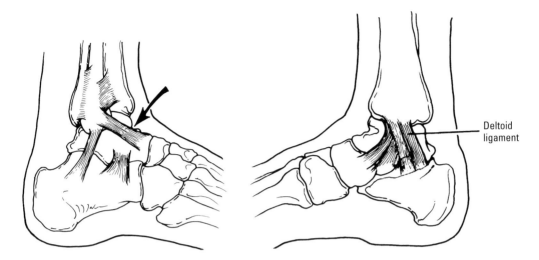

Deltoid
ligament

The ankle.

FIRST AID FOR A SPRAINED ANKLE

1. Ask the casualty to sit or lie down, then support the ankle, trying to find the most comfortable position.
2. Apply an ice pack or ice wrapped in a cloth to the site of the pain, in order to reduce swelling.
3. Gently place soft padding around the ankle, and secure it around the joint with a bandage.

4. Elevate the injured ankle, supporting the weight yourself or on another raised platform.

If you suspect the ankle has been broken, do not move the joint – call for an ambulance or transport the casualty to hospital with the lower limb immobilized. A broken ankle may result in the blood and nerve supply to the foot becoming obstructed. It is therefore

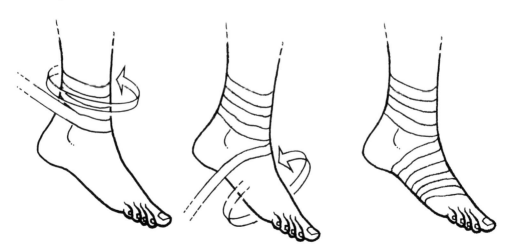

Bandaging the ankle.

123

essential that such an injury is assessed in hospital as quickly as possible.

The martial artist who has suffered a sprained ankle should be advised to see a doctor if the pain and swelling persists for more than a few days.

It is very important to allow a sprained ankle enough time to heal. It may be advisable to seek further medical attention once the pain and swelling have reduced, with regard to a programme of rehabilitation and gradually increasing exercise. A sprained ankle may become prone to injury in the future if it has not been rested sufficiently. It is also advisable to wear an ankle support or to consult a physiotherapist with regard to taping the joint during training. If the injured ankle continues to be unstable, surgical reconstruction of the ligaments may be required.

The Achilles Tendon

The Achilles tendon is the attachment of the calf muscles to the heel bone, or calcaneus. The calf muscles are some of the strongest in the body, and therefore place a considerable amount of strain on this tendon during activities such as running and jumping. As a result, straining of the Achilles tendon is relatively common, and the tendon can also tear, or rupture, completely.

A rupture of the Achilles tendon results in sudden, sharp pain at the back of the heel. The injured martial artist will also be unable to stand on tiptoes, as the calf muscles will no longer be attached to the heel. Such an injury requires urgent medical attention, as prompt surgery is required to prevent loss of function.

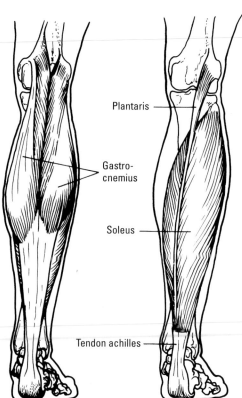

Plantaris

Gastro-cnemius

Soleus

Tendon achilles

The Achilles tendon.

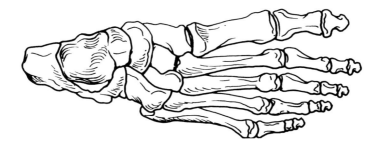

The foot.

Fractures of the Foot

As many martial arts are practised barefoot, the foot is particularly susceptible to injury. The bones of the foot may be fractured as a result of kicking an opponent's elbow, or any other hard surface. Such injuries may be prevented by wearing protective footwear when sparring. The foot is also prone to stress fractures, as a result of training on hard surfaces over long periods of time.

The foot comprises over twenty-five small bones. The heel is formed by the calcaneus, the hindfoot comprises the tarsal bones, and the midfoot is made up of the metatarsal bones. This structure gives the foot both mobility and stability. Each of the toes is also made up of two or three bones. These bones are held together by ligaments, and around many of the joints are fluid-filled joint capsules. Along the sole of the foot, the bones are held in arches. These arches act to absorb some of the forces that are transmitted through the foot, when walking and running.

In the event of a fracture to the foot, the injured person may experience the following features:

- considerable pain;
- difficulty in walking, with the foot being unable to bear any weight;
- rapid swelling and bruising to the area;
- in the case of a fracture of the toe, there may be a distortion in the appearance.

FIRST AID FOR FRACTURES OF THE FOOT
1. Ask the casualty to lie down. Raise the injured foot off the floor and support it on your knees, or on soft padding. This will help to reduce any swelling.
2. Apply an ice pack, or ice cubes wrapped in a cloth, to the site of the pain.
3. Transport the casualty hospital with the foot raised, and with the cold pack still applied.

Blisters

As many martial arts are practised barefoot, blisters on the feet are a relatively common problem. Blisters are the result of excess heat, and in the context of martial arts training, this heat is generated by friction between the foot and the floor. A blister occurs when the top layer of skin separates from the underlying layer, and fluid then begins to collect in the space.

A blister should never be popped or cut, as this will increase the risk of the area becoming infected. Instead, the area should be cleaned and then the pressure taken off the blister by placing a ring-shaped pad around it. If a blister is left to heal of its own accord, the fluid will be absorbed and new skin will grow over the area, without any risk of infection. It is advisable to train wearing sports shoes while blisters are healing.

Bibliography

Books and Resource Packs

First Aid Manual 8th Edition (Dorling Kindersley, 2002)

Archontides, C., Fazey, J. and Smith, N., *Understanding and Improving Skill* (National Coaching Foundation, 1992)

Creager, J. G., *Human Anatomy and Physiology* (Wm. C. Publishers, 1992)

De Vries, M. A., *Physiology of Exercise* (Brown Co., 1986)

Hardy, L. and Fazey, J., *Mental Preparation for Performance* (National Coaching Foundation, 1986)

Hazeldine, R., *Development of Strength and Speed* (National Coaching Foundation, 1985)

Howley, E. T. and Franks, B. D., *Health Fitness Instuctor's Handbook* (Human Kinetics Books, 1992)

Hutson, M., *Sports Injuries Recognition and Management* 3rd Edition (Oxford University Press, 2001)

Kerwin, D., Lindsay, M. and Newton, J., *Introduction to Sports Mechanics* (National Coaching Foundation, 1985)

Lachmann, S., *Soft Tissue Injuries in Sport* (Blackwell Scientific Publications, 1989)

Lamb, D. R., *Physiology of Exercise* (Macmillan Publishing Company, 1984)

McArdle, W. D., Katch, F. I. and Katch, V. L., *Exercise Physiology* (Lea & Fehiger, 1991)

McNaught-Davis, P., *Developing Flexibility* (National Coaching Foundation, 1986)

Norris, C. M., *Sports Injuries Diagnosis and Management* 2nd Edition (Butterworth-Heinemann, 1998)

O'Connor, B., Budgett, R., Wells, C. and Lewis, J., *Sports Injuries and Illnesses* (The Crowood Press, 2003)

Read, M. and Wade, P., *Sports Injuries* 2nd Edition (Butterworth-Heinemann, 2001)

Scottish Sports Council, St Andrew's Ambulance Association and the National Coaching Foundation, *Sports Injury: Prevention and First Aid Management* (Holmes McDougall, 1991)

Sinnatamby, C. S., *Last's Anatomy Regional and Applied* (Churchill Livingstone, 1999)

Wilmore, J. H. and Costill, D. L., *Physiology of Sport and Exercise* (Human Kinetics, 1994)

Woods, B., *Structure of the Body* (National Coaching Foundation, 1986)

Wootton, S., *Nutrition and Sports Performance* (National Coaching Foundation, 1986)

Journals and Magazines

Roosen, A., 'Insight into Thermo-Regulation in Martial Arts', *Traditional Karate* (May 1999)

Terrados, N. and Maughan, R. J., 'Exercise in the heat: Strategies to minimize the adverse effects on performance', *Journal of Sport Sciences* (1995, vol. 13, pp. 55–62)

Thompson, K., 'How to avoid dehydration while competing in Atlanta', *Swimming Times* (May 1996, pp. 28–29)

Wellington, P., 'Fluid facts', *Swimming Times* (August 1994, pp. 24–25)

Index